Dear Gary,
you are so beautiful ...
Blessings,
Cynth
June 2016

Pink Pantie

CONFESSIONS

220 Publishing

Chicago, Illinois
220 Publishing
(A Division of 220 Communications)

by

Cynda Williams

PINK PANTIE CONFESSIONS

Cover Photo by Christina Sanders
Cover Design by 220 Publishing

Published by 220 Publishing
(A division of 220 Communications)
PO Box 8186
Chicago, IL 60680-8186
www.220communications.com
www.twitter.com/220Comm

Williams, Cynda. Pink Pantie Confessions –
ISBN 978-1-5136-0789-4

1. Women's Nonfiction. 2. Self-Help

FOREWORD

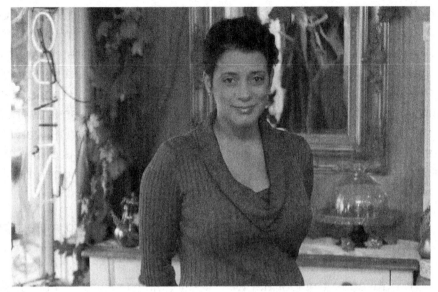

PHOTOGRAPH BY PAUL TROXELL

I have been daring myself to write a book since I was a child. In fact, it was on my bucket list. I was perplexed about what style of book to write since I admired many genres. My mind worked in extremely imaginative ways, so fiction always seemed to be my best bet. Who was going to be my audience? What kind of story would I tell, realistic or fantasy? Although I pondered these questions, I was never able to determine their answers. When I began writing my blog for Pink Pantie Confessions, I tended toward anecdotes, insights, and poetry. After much consideration, I have decided this was as good a place as any to start my literary journey. In fact, this book includes some of my blog and Facebook status posts.

I have an irresistible need to share my thoughts. There is a kind of healing in the action. I kept everything inside and suffered alone through many traumas as a child and through my early adulthood. I believe I became physically and emotionally ill as a result. After surviving surgery, I eventually found the courage to seek help with a psychologist. That two-year "confession" saved my life. From that point on, I began

i

to communicate my feelings as they came to me. Sometimes the outcome was not what I wanted. If someone hurt me, I would tell him or her exactly how I felt, no matter the consequence. Not everyone can handle that kind of honesty. There were times I professed my love, only to be rejected. There has been pain in the telling, but I prefer the truth of my feelings to be out there on the table. That way I can get on with my life regardless of the reaction. These days, if I hold my tongue I become plagued with anxiety. I have to be authentic. I have an immensely negative physical reaction to lying by omission. That doesn't mean I tell every secret. Some truths are classified; meant for me alone or the people I'm experiencing life with. For the most part, I am an open book. I have only a few true friends because of this.

In the early days of my career, fan mail used to come to my agents. That's how I interacted with my supporters. I never invested in a website but instead spent my money in other ways. Thankfully, MySpace was introduced to the world. I was finally able to say "Hi" to the many fans I'd lost contact with over the years. Then Facebook came onto the scene. It took me some time to add this social media giant to my routine but I ultimately signed up, and Facebook became my new way to reach out.

Early on I didn't set up a fan page. I just wanted to communicate personally with these lovely folks; share with them a little of my life. Their support kept me working for so long, I thought it was the right thing to do. Finally, my family and personal friends caught on, so now Facebook has become my primary way of keeping in touch with everyone.

I've expressed myself thoroughly through my statuses. There were times when the ability to vent on my page kept me sane. I have tried to keep my overall viewpoint very positive. When I'm angry, I try to express myself in a way that might help me change my state of mind or help someone else who may be having the same issues. I don't feel so alone when I can tell somebody how I feel. I might be opining about politics or crying over another murder in my home city. I might be demonstrating how to grin and bear it or I might be praising a Good Samaritan. In fact, I often revisit and expand upon my statuses from over the years.

It is my hope that you and I will link together on this journey. My belief is that we are all, every one of us, interconnected through energy exchange. I feel your presence as I write these words. It should be overwhelming, but it is not. I choose to perceive your laughter, tears and understanding. I discern love and companionship in this intimate conversation.

Imagine we are sitting on the deck of a sailboat on a balmy breezy day taking in the rays, drinking Pink Panties (pink lemonade and vodka slushies) and confessing the good moments and the bad.

"Sweetie, let me tell you..."

ACKNOWLEDGEMENTS

I couldn't release this book without acknowledging those that helped me make it happen. I have many people to thank in this first book because IT IS MY FIRST BOOK!

Throughout my life my entire family has supported me. I have had many ups and downs but they have never given up on me. To Charles K. Williams, thank you for giving me a love of books and reading from the start. To Rev. J.C. Williams, Sr. and James "King" Williams thank you for giving me the audacity to write. I watched you over the years modeling myself after you. "If Poppa and King can do it, so can I." I hope I follow in your footsteps. I thank Roderick Plummer for motivating me. He loved to tell me, "Work smart Cindy, not hard." I also want to express gratitude to my brother Charles "Haasan" Williams. He has been there for me since the beginning. Whenever I contemplated quitting any creative effort, he reminded me to "keep the faith."

I want to thank my wonderful contributors Beverly Williams, Lorissa Julianas, Angela Ford, Lynne Hatfield, and Yolanda Harris. I know these shared confessions are but a piece of their great big lives. You are wonderful women and amazing friends.

Without Mike Martin and Shawn Taylor I may never have completed this project. Between our gigs (I sing with his band sometimes) Mike believed in the concept of Pink Pantie Confessions so much he created my blog page without my knowledge. Shawn gave me exceptional advice as we dipped in the Jacuzzi. She suggested I work with 220 Communications, Productions. Munir Muhammed has been an angel for giving me time on his television shows to confess far more openly than some would like. Steven Wolfe of Sneak Preview Entertainment has been more than a professional acquaintance. He has been a phenomenal friend. He makes sure I work! I thank Ken Reynolds of Public Relations+ for taking care of me over the years in so many ways...And for all the fantastic parties, keeping my face in the light.

Thank you, Paul Troxell and Kathleen Mosley for your gift of photography.

I appreciate my blog readers and Facebook friends. You gave me the courage to publish my written words. Stephen Mandel Joseph, William E. Smith, Stephen Stix Josey and James Patterson consistently lifted my spirits with their kind words of encouragement. James has been a great friend in many ways, financially supporting this book, traveling to see my shows and leaving me weekly words of wisdom. I smile every Thursday because of him.

Thank you to Glenn Murray and the 220 Communications team for believing in me from the beginning of this journey. Marisa Anstey helped me enormously. I can be technologically inept and she was gentle with her direction.

A special shout out to Lisa Zure. She opened my eyes to writing with all the senses in mind. Thanks to Joyce Jenkins for diving in and smoothing out my rough edges.

I can't forget my girlz (and one boy pal) on that original Pink Pantie Confession on my 40th birthday. I love you all. You know who you are.

I have "confessed" to my closest friends, Beth Wagner, Anissa Faulkner, Cheryl Youngblood Williams, Robyn Labeaud, Torri Roberts, Peter Bedard, Peter Welz, Thea Camara, and William Lee. I want to particularly thank Deniece "Niece" Payne for being my only true Hollywood actor friend and sister. She introduced me to Pink Panties. I'm not sure if she was the one who created the drink but I always gave her credit. Thank God for my friends. I would have been a total mess without them.

There comes a time in a person's life when everything changes. This last year was that time for me. William Lee (especially), Phylicia Rashad, Yolanda Harris, Beverly Williams, Monica Williams, Sodiqa Williams, Sophia Plummer and Victor Gulley got me through this transition. I will always remember that you were there at my lowest point and helped me out of the darkness and into the light.

Last but most importantly, I have to thank God without whom I would never have had the courage or resilience to start this new journey.

This book is dedicated to my daughter; my love and muse Sophia Gabrielle Plummer.

Contents

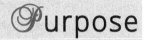

Purpose

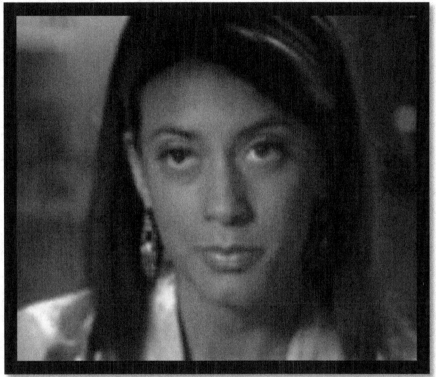

STILL PHOTO FROM 1998 FILM CAUGHT UP

Status:
"Beautiful, Happy, and Successful"
February 19, 2014

A few years ago, I celebrated an important birthday. I am big on birthdays -- I believe in celebrating the life you have been given. Depending on the year, I might find something fun to do for the entire month of May! This specific year I was blessed to be able to take a cruise on *EZ Livin*, my friend's gorgeous bright-white yacht. He was gracious enough

1

to let me have a small group of my closest friends and my family on board. It was a balmy, beautiful day and the shockingly blue ocean rocked the yacht gently as we cruised from Laguna Beach to Long Beach. The cool soothing breeze blew salty Pacific drizzles across my face. I felt a sense of blessed opulence that I'd never known before. It just so happens that most of my chatty friends were female, but I had my closest male partner along also. The captain's exotic Hawaiian missus made delicious finger foods. The savory smells of the islands wafted up and drew me and my friends below. One of my besties had already blended a large crystal pitcher of my favorite drink, Pink Panties. My husband, daughter, and the captain stayed up on deck while the rest of us got to talking down under. It was a four-hour journey I'll never forget.

I'm not sure how it started, but I'm pretty sure it was the sweet and sour drinks. That pink lemonade and vodka started to loosen our tongues and before we knew it we were "confessing" stories from our lives. We were sitting in a circle; it wasn't planned that way but it happened. I believe energy passed from soul to soul that beautiful spring day, a healing energy that we all needed. We began venting about past and present challenges; laughing, crying, cursing and blessing. One friend never said a word, but she was right there with us. Finally, we came to a natural ending of our session. We all sat staring at one another in awe. Then I said, "Pink Pantie Confessions." Someone else said, "This has got to be a book." I said, "...and a movie, TV series, and musical... "

That is when the "Pink Pantie Confessions" odyssey began for me and when the blog started simmering.

It took me awhile to begin the public part of the expedition. I have been writing the musical for some time now (I am a perfectionist). Once I realized the vast opportunities in the web world, I also decided to write "Pink Pantie Confessions" in a web-series format; the numbers I could reach are astounding. Then I realized that women in general are an underserved market. I would never leave out my brothers -- as I've said before, I love men — but they seem to be taking care of themselves. It is time for women to tell their own narratives. Stories are where our spiritual pilgrimages begin. I want to open the door for the truth in those testimonies to be told and shared. When we communicate with each other, the restoration of health begins.

This is an abridged excerpt from the "Pink Pantie Confessions" musical for stage.

Characters: Ruth, Delilah, Sam, Nairobi, and Grace.

Grace and her friends are having a "Pink Pantie Party." They eat nosh, drink Pink Panties, and talk about the past month's challenges. Ruth has brought her much younger sister, Delilah, to the party. Delilah would rather not be there. She seems to be from a different world. The others are self-starters and have a measure of success in their lives. Delilah made dissimilar choices than her sister and is paying for those decisions. It's time for an intervention.

Delilah enters from the bathroom with Ruth close behind.

Ruth: Don't leave sweetie...

Delilah: I've got things to do, Ruth! You can't keep me prisoner here!

Ruth: When you came to me last month, I didn't hesitate to help you. I love you. But there are rules. I told you, you have to stick with me while we figure this all out. You have to be present. No more disappearing acts. Now that we've left the house, you can't wait to bounce. What are you up to?

Delilah: It's none of your business...

Ruth: It became my business when you disrupted my life! (beat) Now sit down and chill out. We're going to be here for a while longer.

Delilah, frustrated and antsy, sits back down.

Ruth: (continuing under her breath) Delilah is beautiful, happy, and successful...

Delilah: Why do you keep talking to yourself? You've done that crap since I could remember. I'm starting to think you're crazy.

The other ladies laugh. Ruth is also tickled.

Ruth: I'm different...Okay, strange, I'll admit.

Sam: I saw you having an animated conversation with yourself a couple of weeks ago. Walking down the street...by yourself...with no phone. You do look crazy.

Grace: Makes me worry...

Ruth: Don't waste your energy! I'm okay. I promise; I've always done it.

Grace: You sure have. Just a lot more lately.

Ruth: I have a very active imagination, that's all. I've always talked to God and myself. Nairobi said it, "Words are very powerful." It's in the Bible, "For if you have faith even as small as a tiny mustard seed you could say to this mountain, 'Move!' and it would go far away. Nothing would be impossible." Matthew chapter 17, verse 20... Daddy's favorite verse. He believed in the power of words, too. That's why I try to stay positive. See, I know I have a gift. I always know what to say to people. I know how to get to them. Read them. I've hurt people when I didn't mean to, though. I've called it speaking the truth, but that can be dangerous. People need to walk their own path, no matter what I think.

Delilah: Yeah; like me.

Ruth: You're different. I've always hesitated to speak to you honestly. You're so sensitive.

Grace: So she's been enabled...

Nairobi: Not anymore. Ruth?

Ruth: No... Not anymore (to Delilah). You want to know why I talk to myself? I'll tell you.

I wanted to be more than the world told me I was capable of. How do you think I've had so much achievement? I speak it, that's how! I found my husband because I saw him in my waking dreams. I imagined his beautiful face. I had conversations with him, out loud, before I ever met him. I melted under his touch, smelled his spicy scent, felt all of him inside my body and my soul then like a miracle; he came to me when I needed him most.

You think my career happened by osmosis? I used to walk Lake Street through downtown looking at all the shops, talking out loud to myself; visualizing, feeling, and hearing the words, "I've made it. I'm the owner of a beautiful boutique and I'm very successful."

Then Grace came to me about her idea for our boutique, Dream Coat. She had a similar dream. I felt those feelings of triumph before the outcome. I met all the important people in my life and had full conversations with them in my mind. I did it unconsciously at first. It came naturally.

Even as a child. I didn't know they were "creative visualizations" until recently when I started reading self-help books after Daddy passed. And that's how I pulled myself up after his death. I talked to myself. It works for me... I see myself as I want to be. I don't dwell on what I fear; I celebrate what God made me: beautiful, happy, and successful.

Ruth sings an exuberant song. Her friends join in the last chorus. Delilah watches somberly.

Beautiful, Happy, and Successful

Verse 1
I'm a glowing, shining light – 'cause I say it
Intelligent and bright – 'cause I affirm it
Bound to win the fight – 'cause I claim it
I will reach my highest height – 'cause I pronounce it
Chorus
I'm beautiful, happy, and successful – Believing is the key
Striking, joyful, and victorious – For all the world to see

Remarkable, blissful, and triumphant – Just like we all can be
Beautiful, happy, and successful – That's what my God made me

Verse 2

I have blessings every day – 'cause I say it
My husband will always stay – 'cause I affirm it
My children will know the way – 'cause I claim it
My God I will obey – 'cause I pronounce it

Chorus

The song ends. Ruth's gladness is contagious. Her friends are almost shouting for joy. Delilah watches sadly.

Status:
"If I touch you, I hope the shattering will set you free."
March 4, 2014

Shattered

Now I know enough to see
Patterns that my life follows
Everything that touches me
Falls apart so quickly
Everything I try to do, or make, or have, or love, or see
Nothing will stay with me
Any friend, or lover, or my home, or my family
I have broken these things so easily
Oh my magic touch shatters everything around me
So if I touch you
I hope the shattering will set you free

Ever since I was a little girl
Everything in my world
In the morning I would have it in my hands, by moonrise it
would blow away like desert sand
Lord tell me that this is not pointless destruction, 'cause I know
that everything must come to pass
I'm just sad because

In my life all I find is made of glass

Lyrics –by Cynda Williams; Music - Cort Fritz

Status:
"Remember."
November 26, 2013

For many years I was very frustrated. You know how you feel when you have an echo of a remembrance tickling your memory? You forget things sometimes and you just can't get the thought back? I walked around constantly trying to remember this something. It was right there on the edge of consciousness. I'd have the slightest twinge of an image and then it was gone. What I was trying to remember was important, but to whom? Could it be the one thought that could shift my trajectory in the right direction?

I made my way through many days with a scowl on my face. The look pasted on my countenance was part conditioning — my father's family tended to frown — and part perpetual wondering. More times than I care to admit, I found myself fighting off angry females who would suddenly yell at me, "Why you glaring at me, bitch?" I'd excuse myself and try to smooth my brow.

It was 3 a.m. Another smoggy Los Angeles morning at my Park Labrea apartment. I lay in my usual state of insomnia. The hunter green paint on the walls of my room made it extremely dark, though a muted gold streetlight streamed in over the slumbering form of my second husband. The smell of Nag Champa incense lingered in the air. I pulled a deep breath into my lungs and tried to meditate, if not sleep. I've always had a difficult time turning off the voices in my head; thinking far too much for my own good. This time was different. There was heaviness in my body. The sensation was foreign and a little frightening. Normal everyday sounds — speeding cars, airplane engines and faraway Jazz riffs — seemed to fade away. The silence became as thick as molasses. I hesitantly opened one watery red-brown eye, then the other. The weighty paralyzing feeling did not subside.

7

An unanticipated movement caught me off guard. I stared in slack-jawed amazement at the far upper right corner of the room. It seemed as if the solid walls were being sucked into the corner and replaced with the vast blackest of black outer space. A million or more stars suddenly appeared. I warily squeezed my eyes shut then opened them again, assuming I had fallen asleep, into an incredible dream. No, I was awake. I'm not stupid. My fifth grade school teacher taught me that stars are large balls of gas that would burn the Earth up in a flash if they got near enough. These humongous suns are really millions of miles away. But the corner of my bedroom ceiling looked like the night sky after I'd traveled a few hundred miles away from L.A. into the Sedona desert.

The celestial bodies seeped from the corner, filling the room surrounding me. "Dang! What in the H-E double hockey sticks am I seeing?" I tried to move my leaden form but couldn't. I thought, "Am I dying or finally going out of my freakin mind?"

I'd read lots of sci-fi in my day, so I knew that whenever the "grey" aliens came to visit someone, the person might be unable to move. They endured a loss of control of their motor muscles. Was I going to have a close encounter of the third kind? I had no desire to see some naked, bald, big-eyed thing next to my bed. I heard a whisper in my right ear. "Remember?"

Ahhh, man.

"Go away!" I thought as loudly as I could, since I could not muster the will to physically speak. "I don't want to know what you are and I won't go to your spaceship with you. I have to get my rest. I have an audition tomorrow. So what if it's for a part in a sitcom playing a hoochie mamma again? I need the money!"

I got no response so I continued searching for the invading grey aliens. Or might they be the vicious insectiles? Reptilians? God help me. Nothing but sparkling stars still floated above. All of a sudden, the stars whooshed away toward the right upper corner and out of the room at a single point. I was left in complete darkness. No more warm, slightly musky, husband next to me, no more California king-sized bed that swallowed us up. No more me. But my thoughts were still there and I could physically feel with my mind. I felt a density in the darkness. I perceived weight, as if my spirit was draped in black billowing velvet drapes. The voice whispered again. "Remember." And then I did. I was in a familiar place: my mother's womb, warm and safe. Waiting. I'd been there before. The voice asked, "Are you ready for your journey? You have all the tools you need to learn all your lessons of this life. Are you ready?" I answered, "Yes." And I was. The voice flitted away; the walls of my room blew back into place. Peaceful bliss enveloped me, more profound than anything I'd ever felt before. I finally remembered the memory that had always teased me. I wasn't sure of the answer I gave while in the womb, but I knew now for certain, that there was someone outside of myself that cared to know. And I also knew that there is a reason for me being here. All the trials ARE for something. I looked at my snoring partner and smiled. I usually told him everything, but not this time. His sleep needed not be disturbed. This serene moment was mine and my awe exceeded my fear.

PINK PANTIE
CONFESSIONS

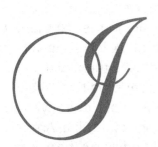

*I*dentity

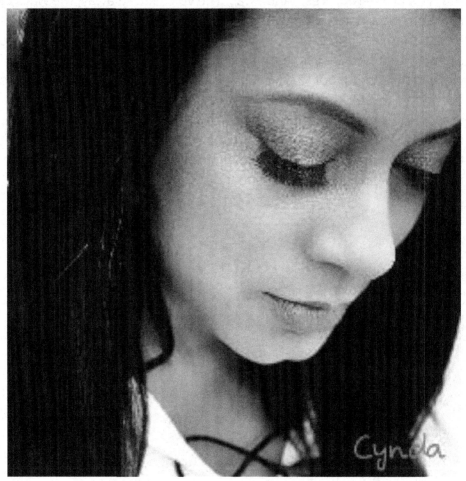

PHOTOGRAPH BY KATHLEEN MOSLEY

Status:
"Dig deep and look inside."

"Who am I? I'm growing every day into who I am – not what I do or whose I am. I've got to trust that who I am today is enough. I love who I am."

I posted this on my Facebook and Twitter pages recently for a reason. My sister Sodiqa had been trying to get me to read Neale Donald Walsh's, "The Only Thing That Matters – Book Two in the Conversations with Humanity." I'd read many of Neale's books, but it had been awhile. They had been life-altering reads.

I believed 2014 has the potential to be a transformational year, so I decided I was ready to take another personal journey with Neale. Then I realized Sodiqa skipped his first book in the series: "The Storm Before the Calm – Book One in the Conversations with Humanity." Did I mention that I tend to be extremely neat and organized? I couldn't possibly start with Book Two — that would be out of order. (I sometimes laugh at myself about this trait and am determined to work on this; I'm way too attached to supposed 'order.')

In his book, Neale poses some very challenging questions, although they seem to be simple. One question he suggested we ask ourselves is, "Who am I?" No big deal, right?

I sat in my office ruminating on this question for a long time before I could admit some honest truths to myself. Gazing from my vision boards of the past and present to my spiritual artwork adorning the walls, I realized that I so often think of "me" in terms of what I do. Neale didn't ask, "What do you do?" or "What do others say?" Spending so much time doing and so little time being, I had no idea who the hell I was! I'd always tried to make things happen, never trusting that I am exactly where I'm supposed to be. I feared living in the moment. By imposing my immovable will, I've never fully succeeded. Forcing life to listen to me, or else, doesn't work. Why do you think I'm always coming up with self-motivating thoughts? I'm trying to get past belief and KNOW that I am blessed, abundant, and successful, right now.

11

This is who I think I am today: I am a sometimes-conscious being. I am a seeker of truths. I am a student of the universe. I am a teacher. I am an artist. I have been given the gift of inspiring moods, thoughts, and feelings in others by using creative expressions inspired by something bigger than me with my words, voice, and imitation of life. Who I am affects others directly and indirectly.

Am I living my life with "who I am" in mind? Are my choices reflecting who I am? I believe so. Even the so-called mundane experiences of day-to-day living — paying bills, cleaning, cooking, eating, working, and relating — have taught me how to better be who I am. How "am I" when I do these things? I try to pay attention to every detail of every act. When I cut onions I allow the tears to cleanse me of whatever I might need to release. When I pay my bills I stay thankful for yet another month of income to take care of my responsibilities. When I drive to the corner store I smile at the other drivers and may even wave. When I wake up in the morning I step outside to speak to all the flying and creeping creatures. When I tuck my daughter in for bed I praise my higher being for the gift of this sweet young lady. When I take a walk I celebrate that I can walk. When the computer freezes I say thank you to the universe for the siesta that I need. Of course you know I am nothing like perfect. Not even close. I have to remind myself continuously to delight in the small lessons and big challenges.

There is so much to ponder in that simple question, "Who am I?" I will be answering it every day.

Happy 2014, my friends. Let's all dig deep and look inside. We can change the world starting today.

Status:
"It's really cool when you come to your senses."
April 11, 2014

Came To My Senses

I make this promise to you
I saw gray skies and assumed they were blue

12

I never truly knew
My lying brain wasn't true
Until I came to my senses
You've got to know
That I always felt low
So low, I couldn't grow
The brilliant sun didn't glow
Until I came to my senses
I swear to my God
I felt my heart flawed
My love was a fraud
I thought ardor odd
Until I came to my senses
I assure you, I'm real
That I didn't feel
Until I started to heal
And live life with zeal
That's when I came to my senses

Status:
"Fear is the antithesis to love."
March 11, 2014

We Williamses were apartment dwellers for the first five years of my life. West Side Chi-town! I don't remember much of that time. There are flashes of recollection: some extended family gatherings, my pretty towering five foot two mother chasing me around the dingy apartment with a reeking fish head, my Uncle King's flashy multi-colored bell-bottom jeans and diamond studded vests, a birthday party for my brother Haasan, my father's disk-shaped bloodshot eyes as he laughed loudly at a joke I didn't understand.

The first fleshed-out remembrances of my early childhood start in 1972 when we moved to 10431 South King Drive. Our very own house! I was absolutely enthralled with our two-story red brick house. I remember running through the three large bedrooms trying to decide which one was going to be mine. The roomy master was my first choice but, of course, my parents had the nerve to claim it.

Being the only girl child, I was the only family member that didn't have to share so I was issued the tiniest treasure. It was said that the original owner built this room for his daughter, so it was perfect. My lovely light-filled bedroom faced the lush backyard. The two large windows allowed me to all but live in the trees. My favorite was the Evergreen tree. I imagined Christmas was everyday as I sniffed the flaky bark and watched the squirrels and birds eat the seeds. Being a loner, I spent most of my time reading, singing, hoping and dreaming in my simple space. It could be messy in there but it was mine.

The only full bath was enormous. I spent many nights dozing in the large mint green porcelain glazed tub. My brothers loved to bang on the door to scare me from my stupor. The half bath on the main floor served several purposes. Relief and clean hands were two, but also closeted cigarette smoking. My parents never got away with it though. I would lay down and stick my nose under the door saying, "I smell that Mommy. You're smoking and I know it Daddy! You're going to die if you don't stop smoking!"

In winter my father, brothers and I cuddled with hot chocolate in front of the large fireplace in the sparse living room/family room. Family photos lined the ledge of the mantle. The white walls remained empty in the beginning. It took a while to fill up all that space. We watched many sports events on our small black and white. My dearest spot in there was the picture window overlooking the busy street. I wondered where all those people were rushing off to.

For a while, our dining room remained empty but it would eventually hold a long formal table for twelve. There were built-in maple cabinets holding our family heirlooms. My favorite room, the kitchen, was where we spent much of our time. It was bright and yellow with orange splashes so I always felt happy while we ate our meals, did our homework and talked from morning to night around the kitchen table.

Our basement was finished. Daddy eventually put a pool table down there. I enjoyed watching many a tension-filled game unfold between Daddy and his police friends. They would always end with a drink and a laugh.

There was nothing like exploring the largest back yard on the block (or at least it seemed that way to me). I communed with bouncing rabbits, fearless squirrels, regal cardinals and spirited blue jays as I climbed the five towering trees. There was a spruce, a pine, a crabapple and a maple tree. I imagined I was Snow White deep in the forest. So plentiful was the yard space that we could have had half the neighbors over for a party. Eventually we often did that, but not that summer. When we first moved in, my brothers were still little bitties. Fred was barely born and Haasan would more likely eat worms than bother with me so I played alone. Oddly, the quiet neighborhood seemed void of children. Obviously people lived in the other houses because when I walked by them I would see hands yanking the drapes closed. This was strange because it was in the middle of a hot, muggy summer. Why weren't other kids outside frolicking in the sunshine? There were rejected barbeque grills in the other yards, even some pools, but no one attended them. Therefore, I was lonely. Assuming incorrectly that moving into a neighborhood meant having neighborhood friends, I was disheartened by my unending solitude.

 Finally my luck changed. One day as I played pretend out back, I noticed a little girl about my age walk into her backyard from her house two doors down. I was so excited, I *knew* there had to be kids! There were steel wire fences and another house separating us, but I didn't care. I called over and introduced myself. The girl was as beautiful as a Renaissance portrait. Twisting her red curly ringlets that fell to her lower back, she timidly spoke to me. She said she had been indoors all summer and was just tired of it, so she snuck outside while her mother washed clothes.

That was the beginning of a sweet friendship. I wanted to go to her house or have her come to mine, but the girl discarded the idea. She wasn't supposed to be outside, remember? For five blissful days I played with that girl from afar; we giggled, told secrets, spoke of dreams. This was the energy exchange I'd been craving, although I was never quite satiated. It was never longer than a half an hour before the girl had to go back inside to her prison. I felt sorry for her.

On day six everything changed. As we spoke over the fences of our escapades the night before, a young, rusty, freckled-faced man came outside. He smiled benevolently at his daughter. But then he looked at me. His demeanor changed so suddenly, I panicked. Looking around to make sure no monsters were in sight, I became confused. He was visibly upset as he regarded his daughter then re-entered the house. My friend knew she had done something wrong. She just wasn't sure what. Moments later, her young pretty blond pixie of a mother came out. She did not look my way; would not. It was as if her fairy life depended on it. She quietly reprimanded her daughter as she forcibly yanked her into the house. I was dumbfounded. What just happened? I wasn't the type of kid to ask my parents. They seemed so overwhelmed by life that I kept my problems to myself. I went to bed that night in tears.

The next day I came outside to look for my friend. She didn't come out. I waited all day for her, waited several days before I gave up. I started playing inside in my room because I was depressed. As someone who felt things very deeply, I had many sleepless nights because I over processed. I wanted to understand, how could something so right turn into something so wrong?

Two weeks later, I began feeling more like myself. Adoring trees, I decided it was time to climb one. The maple tree was my best friend; he would lift me high to see my new world from above. I scrambled up to the top of my tree and quietly took it all in. That's why she didn't see me when she came outside. I realized that she looked for me. When she was sure I wasn't present, she began to play in the grass. She rolled down the slight hill breathing in the musty soil. As I called her name, her startled baby blues ascended the tree to where I straddled a thick gnarly limb. She peered back at her house with trepidation. Motioning for me to "shush" she blushed in apparent discomfiture. My friend continued to frolic in the lawn. She never looked at me as she answered

16

my questions. "Where have you been?" I asked. She said, "In the house most of the time. Mommy and Daddy said I couldn't play with no niggers." "What's a nigger?" I inquired. She said, "I don't know what it means but that's what you are, I think. My daddy said you and your daddy are black so that makes you niggers." I said, "I don't get it." She impatiently said, "Your skin is black, Cindy. That makes you a nigger." I looked at my friend, and then examined myself. I didn't see much of a difference. "I'm not black. I'm cream like for coffee. My daddy's brown like a dark chocolate Hershey and my mommy's peach...like you. Not the orange skin but the inside meat." She continued to scrutinize the blades of grass she yanked out at the roots, but I saw the bewilderment on her face. "That's true. I am peach. I don't know," she said, "But my family can't stay here no more. The niggers are moving in and you're one of them. Niggers are bad and lazy. They'll ruin the neighborhood. That's why we're moving. Everybody is."

I turned and noticed the moving truck in front of her house. It wasn't the first I'd seen. I contemplated my friend one last time. She finally took me in with a small, sad smile. "Cindy, I'm going to miss my house. And you. You sure are a nice nigger. You don't seem all that scary to me. I don't see what the big deal is." She rose and forlornly dragged her feet into her house, leaving me with my first realization that I was different and to be feared. Wow. I was very powerful if my skin could scare a whole neighborhood into moving out of their gorgeous homes. Niggers are mighty strong.

ℕucleus

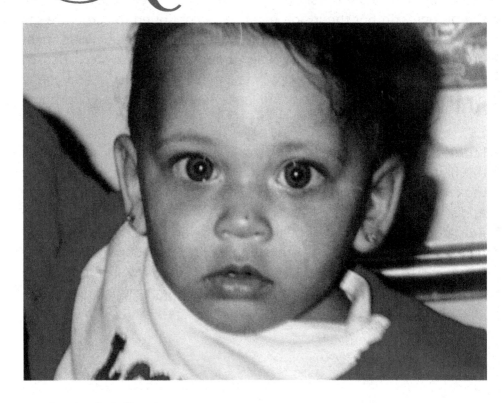

Sophia Gabrielle Plummer

Status:
"Dare to be Different."
November 25, 2013

This morning my daughter was going through her typical school-day morning ritual. She got up, washed her face, brushed her teeth, and TRIED to get dressed. No matter if she sets her clothes out the night before, Sophia invariably changes her mind over and over again about what she is going to wear. Usually her choices are based on her Converse color moods. Does she feel like coral, pink, or black? Green, teal blue, or aquamarine? On basketball game days, the dayspring journey is even more perilous. Her team is required to dress up. No athletic shoes, no jeans. She hates those days. Sophia is truly a jeans and t-shirt type.

This morning the problem was shoes. My daughter could not decide which shoes to wear. She doesn't have many. Her feet have grown so quickly it's hard to keep her in them, but she's got a few. She moans, "It's cold outside. I don't have nice boots."

Now I know that to be false. Sophia has at least two pairs of boots. They both have a 2-inch heel but they are nice. Last year she loved them (thankfully I bought them up a size). This morning she said, "They make me too tall. I'm already taller than everyone else! I don't want to wear heels anymore." By that she meant, taller than the boys. I remember that's how I felt at her age. I asked Sophia why she cared. She answered me with these oh so common, heart wrenching words, "I want people to like me."

Wow... I stared at her for an unusually mute moment, mouth hanging open. I couldn't understand this conversation. My beautiful baby was standing there, beat down? Believing in her heart that being taller than others meant she wouldn't be liked. I've always encouraged my daughter and pointed out her strengths. She is intelligent, kind, generous, well-behaved and striking. She has long, shapely legs, the perfect behind (Brazilian babes beware), an exotic countenance, sandy brown full hair, and the most piercing green eyes. Consistently, I've praised her while trying to help her grow through her weaknesses. I thought I'd always bolstered her confidence. Man. The preteen years can throw all that parenting out the window!

I eventually asked her to "Dare to be different. Being confident in your differences is what will attract people to you."

This conversation took me back to when I was Sophia's age. I was a very shy child. I'd experienced traumatic events in my life. These occurrences shaped me into a friendless, somber, soft-spoken person. I had little to no self-esteem. I believed I was the most hideous person on Earth.

What made matters worse? My teeth. When I began getting my permanent teeth they came in cracked and with little enamel. I'm not sure what the disease is called, but it made my already sad self even more mournful. I could not smile without exposing the decay-filled cracks in my teeth. There was no toothbrush to get into those hairline fissures so I had cavities in the front of my smile. My parents at the time couldn't afford the deductible to pay a dentist. I just covered my mouth with my hand and kept it shut. It was terrible.

One day I'd had enough. I was in sixth grade; near to the age my daughter is now. I decided I wasn't going to allow my past and my teeth to stop me from having friends and fun. I'll never forget it. We had a Christmas party. The customary slightly stinky smell of children's body odor, chalk, and disinfectant was replaced by the fragrance of sugar cookies. Merry, colorful, urchin holiday art covered the walls. My teacher sat at her desk watching us with a smirk as we grooved to The Commodores crooning out of the record player speakers. All of my classmates were dancing and laughing and I was doing what I always did: sitting in a corner reading a book. I was so envious of the joy I saw on their faces. Everyone had his or her differences. There were heavy kids, kids with thick glasses, kids with knobby knees, kids with ashy elbows, kids with braces, kids with worn clothes, kids with smelly armpits. Kids -- all wonderful uniquely different kids. I decided right there and then, "No more!" They can laugh at my ugly mouth all they want to. They can make fun of me. I'm going to have fun and SOMEBODY is going to like me. SOMEBODY is going to be my friend! That decision changed my life. I got up and started dancing like I'd done in the quiet of my bedroom for years. My classmates were shocked. They'd never seen this Cindy and they liked her! I made lifelong friends that day.

I told my daughter that story. I hope she decides to embrace her differences and love herself. Because it ain't no lie — If you don't love yourself exactly as you are, no one else EVER will.

Status:
"My Dear."
April 8, 2014

I wrote these lyrics for my daughter when she was born. My friend Phil Gardenhire wrote the music far before he met me. It is one of my favorite songs of any I've penned. I will record it soon.

My Dear

When I look into your eyes
I see blue stars flit by
When I feel your warm embrace
I thank Him the Most High
Cause now I know what love's about
Now I know its face

Come with me for all time
Be with me always
Come and hold your hand in mine
In nighttime and my days

Cause now I know what love's about
Cause now I know its face
It's you my dear
Lyrics by Cynda Williams; Music by Phil Gardenhire

Status:
"Do Unto Others."
March 24, 2014

My daughter and I had a day that is worthy of note.

Sophia was called in at the last minute to be an alternate in a special game for her basketball league. The situation was bittersweet because she knew that if other teammates had been available for the entire game she would not have been given a second thought. I tried to help her understand that the world often times worked that way. You aren't always the "chosen one" (don't I know that!). By the time we arrived to the game, I think I had her convinced that being selected was the blessing. In any case, inside the sticky gym we came upon the three "chosen" girls preparing for the one quarter they were to play. These lovely little ladies COMPLETELY ignored my daughter. It was as if she didn't exist. This was nothing new. These three had been very condescending to the other players on the team the entire season. They had become a three-girl squad. See, they'd received intensive training and playing time because of their last year; their skills had excelled beyond the rest of the team. The remaining, less-experienced girls had natural talent, but for one reason or another (most usually expense), they did not receive that extensive instruction. The regrettable thing was, two of the girls were easily engaging with their teammates the year before. But their new-found proficiency and alliance to the leader of their little pack tainted their nature. I hoped this behavior would be short-lived. They were good girls at heart. In the meantime, Sophia was devastated by their rejection. She had the "only child" fantasy of being friends with everyone. As she quaked in irritation and humiliation, I told her that just because she had to work with these girls did not make them her friends. Their behavior made them unworthy of her companionship. She went on to do her best in the game. Unfortunately, her team was not as prepared as the other, so they lost.

I wanted to cheer my daughter up so I took her to a little cafe for lunch after the game. It wasn't fancy, but I thought a fun meal of hotdogs and French fries could raise her spirits. We were the only customers except for one table of young men. They were about 18-20 years old. They guffawed and shoved large portions of food down their throats. While we waited for our meals to arrive, a scruffy man in his seventies came in and sat down. I believe he worked in the kitchen. He was obviously tired and a little down and out. Seemingly lonely, he waited for a cab to arrive. For some reason, he decided to start a conversation with the young men.

His voice was very loud and caused the guys to cringe. The elder started talking about how difficult the streets of Chicago seemed. He wanted to discuss his family and friends. One or two of the young men decided to be respectful and participated in a back and forth with the gentleman. Suddenly, the second comrade, uninterested and bothered, decided enough was enough. "We're trying to eat here! Leave us alone!" The first guy who had shown some benevolence was stunned into silence. Sophia and I couldn't believe his rudeness. The old man stopped talking and stared at his blemished, hardened hands. I wanted to say something, but the man had not engaged me. It didn't seem appropriate. The aged man's cab arrived and he despondently shuffled out of the restaurant. The arrogant man-child began to laugh, unfeelingly. The others scolded him, but it was too late.

My sensitive daughter lost her appetite. She asked to leave immediately as her full bottom lip quivered and she held back mournful tears. She felt the pain of dismissal right along with the grandfather. She'd only just encountered her own rejection that morning, so she empathized. "How can people be so mean?" she asked.

I didn't know. I don't know now. It seems so simple to show a little mercy. You never know whose life you are affecting when you demonstrate the slightest compassion. The three arrogant girls and the ignorant young man had no sense of consideration. It made me wonder if they had any home training. These days it seems kids are not taught, 'Do unto others as you would like them to do unto you.' I hope that old man went home, hugged his wife, and went on with his day. My instinct told me something different.

Sophia and I rode home in silence. I eventually told her something like this, "Take what happened today as a lesson in how NOT to be to people. If your skills excel beyond others', show thoughtfulness always. Remain humble. Say hello. Have a kind word. You don't know who this person might be in your life. They might end up being your best friend or your boss one day. If an elder or one less fortunate talks to you with earnestness, it can't hurt you to respectfully listen. You may one day grow old or lonely and need the company of strangers."

I believe in Karma. You do reap what you sow, the positive and the negative. Maybe not right away, but life has a way of reminding you of your deeds.

Sophia and I went home, held each other, and prayed for our world.

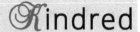

Kindred

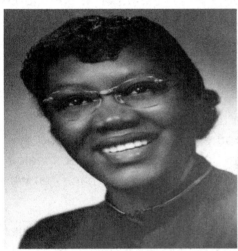
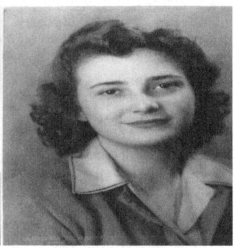

Rosa Mae Williams   Eula Swartz

Status:
"Been thinking about my Grandmas."
March 4, 2014

Grandmothers can be very special. The images of them on television and in the movies portray nurturing, warm, white-haired fountain-heads of wisdom. I think we realize that these representations are the archetype and not necessarily the norm.

My grandmothers were very distinctive women. Though they both were strong matriarchal figures in their families, they were always develop-ing. They were flawed like we all are. While they were coming up as young women, the United States was a different place. They both had to overcome major disadvantages and cultural mores that are unpopular today.

Rosa Mae Williams

Grandma (Paris) Williams was a pillar of strength in her community. All people respected her. She was beautiful and solid as a rock. You always knew what you were getting when you asked her opinion; she never pulled punches. Grandma was also an unsympathetic disciplinarian. She rarely smiled (as a matter of fact, she frowned constantly) and scared many young kids. My grandma was the mother of our church and took her job very seriously. I modeled many aspects of my life after her. I feared and loved her very much. Grandma educated me in many ways. She taught me how to clean thoroughly. I learned the basics of cooking. Grandma was an amazing cook. She was very crafty and had a green thumb. My aunt often tells me how much like her I am. It is a great compliment to me. Grandma trained me how to work hard for what I wanted. I knew my grandmother cared for me even though I don't remember her ever saying she loved me. She did not speak in clichés. She just took time to teach me how to be a woman. That was love in action.

I used to wait until Grandma Williams came to visit to get sick. It's like my body knew she would take care of me. She never was kindly while she assisted me through my ailments. She was rational and direct. "Lay down." "Blow your nose." "Take your cod liver oil." She did not tuck me in lovingly. That wasn't her way but she was there for me when I needed her most. She did not hesitate to take a switch to my bottom if she believed I was behaving badly.

One time I was having tea with her. I hit the side of my teacup a few times with my dainty spoon as I stirred the honey inside. Grandma Williams slapped me so hard I had a handprint across my face. She did not play. This was the way she was raised to bring up children. She bore severe punishment as she grew up so she doled it out without a blink. She not only whipped my butt but all my siblings, cousins, and the church children she thought were being disobedient.

My Grandmother Williams never gave me compliments. She often made unkind comments. She was the epitome of truthful. She had no filters; she told you what she thought no matter how harsh. As I grew older I began to question her love. I often wondered If she liked me. After I moved away to New York and started a life of my own, I would come back to Muncie to visit my family. Grandma suffered many ailments. She had glaucoma, high blood pressure, and several strokes. I made sure I spent time with her. My great-grandmother died at a young age and I wanted to make sure I had memories that would last all the way until the end. Our relationship changed when I asked my grandmother, "Why don't you like me? Why do you say such mean things?" Grandma paused and I could see the shock on her face. She asked me what I meant and I explained my feelings. She told me then and there, "I love you, Cindy, just like I love all of my grandchildren. If I say something to offend you, you have to speak up. I don't always say what I mean to completion. If you don't talk to me, I won't know. I don't want to hurt you." I will never forget that conversation. It was a blessed gift. She passed pretty soon after that. It took me a couple of years to really mourn her. I felt it was my duty to keep the family uplifted in and around her death. She was the glue that kept us together. When I grieved her, I felt like my heart was being squeezed and torn apart. I mended, but I still miss her. I am thankful to have had her in my universe.

Eula (Dennie) Swartz

Grandma Swartz was a tough, loyal, and striking woman. She was a tower of strength in her small community. Grandma Swartz was very outspoken about her beliefs in church, God, and her country. My mother Beverly was her first child. Mommy contracted polio and Grandma made sure my mother was taken care of. She didn't take the doctor's word that my mom was going to die a terrible death, be a vegetable, or never function in life. She fought to give her daughter all the tools she needed to have a full proactive life. She also took care of her two other children and loved her husband. She was active in the church and worked a full time job at the post office.

When my grandfather Albert tragically died with his brother–in-law in a plane accident, Grandma had to again show her sturdiness. She could not break down and give up. She had to continue on. It was no matter that she carried a heavy load alone. My mother was 18 when her dad died. She and Grandma suffered with the loss. They began to receive counseling from my pastor grandfather, Rev. J.C. Williams. That is how my parents met and where the conflict with my grandmother and mother began. Fortunately, Grandma met a wonderful widower with three children and remarried. They raised their children with love. But Mommy was not living her life in the way they deemed proper. When she and my dad started dating, Grandma put her out.

I believe Grandma Swartz thought she was being righteous. Whites and blacks could break bread together, even pray together, but NEVER marry. That was how she was raised in Parker, Indiana. Grandma and Grandpa tried to accept my parents' union, so they struggled with it. Still, my grandmother remained a mysterious being to me and my brothers. Every once in a while they would show up at our home in Chicago. These visits were short but sweet. I remember the sounds of soft conversation, the smell of coffee by 4:30 a.m., and the reluctant hugs. Grandma never hesitated to smile. Her smile was beatific and shined a light on the confusing stopovers.

Very often my father, mother, siblings, and I would take road trips to Muncie, Indiana to visit the family. Grandma and Poppa Williams were very busy with Trinity Church. They had a proactive social agenda so they couldn't visit us in Chicago too often. We'd see them and then go to visit our other grandparents. Those trips were often uncomfortable. There was an unseen oppressive energy whenever we made an appearance at their house. My father always seemed to be on the defensive. He remained prepared to pounce with any provocation. I didn't know who the enemy was. In spite of this, I enjoyed my time there. I loved watching their interactions with each other. They were so easy going. I always wanted to be in on the joy.

I had a couple of run-ins with a cousin. Up to that point I had only experienced direct racism once when I was five years old. My cousin enjoyed calling us "niggers." He hated us, and I didn't know why. We were family, right? He always got disciplined so I decided he was just "not a nice kid." I'd run into nasty children before. It didn't occur to me that he had to have learned that behavior from somebody.

These clandestine visits went on for years. When I turned 13 everything changed. I was in Muncie for the summer but I hadn't seen much of the Swartzes. My friend was a cheerleader for Parker High School and invited me to come to the parade. She suggested that we could surprise my grandparents after. The idea excited me. I couldn't wait to see the looks on their faces when I popped over. I wrote a song to immortalize the event. Here are the lyrics.

Lulla "bye"

Sing to me Grandmother a lulla "bye," it's good to be with you tonight
But before you go tell me why your skin has no color?
And the old woman doesn't answer the question asked in innocence

The love of a child is simple and carefree
There's no love in an old woman afraid (ashamed) of what she sees in me

I thought I'd surprise you
So one day after school
I found myself in front of your house not knowing it was too soon
A few of my dreams and all of my pride
Would be gone as soon as I rang the bell, but you wouldn't let me inside

Day turns to night
And finally you ask me by

But when the sun brings back the light
I'll take my face away from you and find a place to hide

If somehow you hear this, well I guess you already knew
You only hurt me because I loved you
They say that love is blind don't we wish that were true
All I know is that love needs courage inside of me and inside of you

The love of children is simple and carefree
That's the kind of love I want inside of me
Day turns to night
And finally you ask me by
But when the sun brings back the light
I'll take my face away from you and find a place in the light

I will never forget the looks on their faces as I stood there pleading to be let into the screen door. It dawned on me as I stood there that I had never been to their house unless it was dark. I became so angry, I had to turn around and leave as soon as possible. My friend (who was white) was mortified. It took me a long while to get over that snub from these people whom I thought adored me. But truly they never treated my brothers and I the same as they did their other grands. We were aliens to their world. We were tolerated for blood's sake but the stigma of racism was hard to break through. I'm sure they thought they were protecting us. If the neighbors and the extended family knew we existed, we may have experienced a lot worse than my cousin's wrath. I can't help thinking they were shielding themselves more.

Time went on and my grandparents evolved. When my sisters were born, enough time had passed to loosen up the ties of bigotry. It also helped that we had moved to the nearby town. They had time to get to know my sisters and love them with a passion. Honestly, I was envious of the relationship my sisters had with them. It took me a while to mature enough to understand the growth that was occurring. My grandmother always stuck to certain right-wing, religious conservative beliefs, but she realized that it was not 'Christ-like' to mistreat people, especially her progeny.

After Grandpa Swartz passed, Grandma and I gradually came together. She often wrote me letters. She seemed to be proud of me. She even took to boasting to other family members about my successes. What I loved the most about her was, she never stopped loving and supporting my mother. Grandma took care of my mother until her own passing. I always appreciated her loyalty. She ended her journey by voting for Barack Obama. She had grown that much.

I was blessed to have my grandmas. I now understand that they did the best that they could do while here on this plane. They were great then and I believe greater now. I still feel their presence. I believe they help me with difficult choices. I hope to have my own grandchildren one day. I hope they can look past my flaws and relish all the love I have to give them. That is my prayer.

Status:
"I stop...and breathe...I flow through the unseen spaces when my own skewed perception blocks me."
June 14, 2013

Fascinating

Sitting in the park one day,
I saw a sight that took me by surprise.
I still can't fathom how I felt that way
Considering my heart was cold as ice.

His laughing voice absorbed all my pain
Loving caring for his children on his own.
Watching carefree games I was so entertained
I wondered why his woman let him do it all alone.

Fascinating.
He's fascinating

So fascinating to me.
Fascinating
He's fascinating,
He's fascinating to me.

Enticing me with gentle tones and quiet ways
I was mystified by every word.
Electrified when I heard him say,
"Mommy went to Heaven like a bird."

It's too soon to want him
It's too soon to act
I know I can't have him
So I'll have to go back.
And when he is ready
I'll be there it's true
And I am sure I will fascinate him too.

Lyrics by Cynda Williams; Music by Phil Gardenhire

Status:
Saturday Chores Fantasy
December 3, 2014

I was six years old. It was Saturday at 7 a.m. Mommy, Haasan, Frederick and I already had breakfast. Daddy went to his CPD patrol as soon as he swallowed down his black coffee. We always rose early in those days. Crispy bacon, fried eggs, toast and buttered "Wonder Bread" filled our teeny bellies and readied us for our ritual of morning chores. Mommy and Daddy had me working as soon as I could walk. Every Saturday I was in charge of vacuuming. I would push and pull that massive, loud contraption through our cranberry shag carpet, loving life. This was my favorite time of the week because it was when I could dream up all kinds of situations so clearly and in peace. I'd speak out loud for every character in my fantasy. The vacuum gave me all the privacy I needed. I'm sure my Mommy listened and watched at times but her furtive looks didn't bother me. The day's fantasy was exciting:

I was sitting in the front and center of my cramped first grade class-room. All my feisty classmates were still agitated because of some drama outside at recess. That's the way it was every day. Always some drama... Maybe Jennie and Belinda got in another fight. They fought all the time. Or maybe Trenton was doing back flips again; or John-John showed some girl his thing. Boy, was he nasty. I was excited because I did very well in the double-dutch competition.

You know this was a fantasy! In reality, I was always hiding in a corner of the playground. I was so shy. I had no friends and I could barely jump with a single rope; talk about clumsy. But in my vision I was a "bad" with the double-dutch.

The classroom smelled of perspiration and Lysol. But I was cool and composed. I was dressed in my favorite hand-me-down jeans with nee-dlepoint flowers down the thigh (I sewed those myself), striped red, white and blue t-shirt and my moon shoes.

I smiled because I was happy. Very happy. The room went quiet and I noticed the ever jovial Mrs. Brown standing in front of the class. Her presence was phenomenal.

Mrs. Brown commanded respect in her quiet and kind way. Everyone at Bennett Elementary loved her. She was huge and I constantly imag-ined all that girth wrapped around me in a tight hug.

Mrs. Brown wore a beautiful flowered dress that fit her 220-pound body in all the right places, brown face glowing. She beamed at me, holding several pieces of papers in her hand. She said, "Class, I am very proud of most of you; those of you who did your writing assignment." She looks very pointedly at a couple of students. They dropped their heads in shame. "Most of you made a true effort in writing your poetry. There are a couple of students that stand out. Cindy, I'd like you to read your poem to the class." I couldn't believe it! I got to read my poem! In front of everyone! I liked performing for others.

So I read aloud:

"Teacher

Every day that you smile

It makes me happy to be with you for just a while.

Means the world to me, Teacher"

With tears in her eyes, Mrs. Brown said, "Cindy, I love your poem. It means so much to me. Thank you."

I said, "Thank you, Mrs. Brown."

Tracey, who sat behind me, whispered, "You're such a teacher's pet."

"No I'm not." I answered confidently. "I don't care what you think. Just because you're not the one getting attention, don't be mean to me."

Mrs. Brown, having heard the entire exchange, said, "That's enough girls. You're both very talented and smart, too. Tracey, I want to hear your poem next."

Tracey stuck out her tongue at me and I just laughed. My feelings are not hurt one bit.

I vacuumed on as all of this plays in my mind and the words trickle off my tongue.

PINK PANTIE
CONFESSIONS

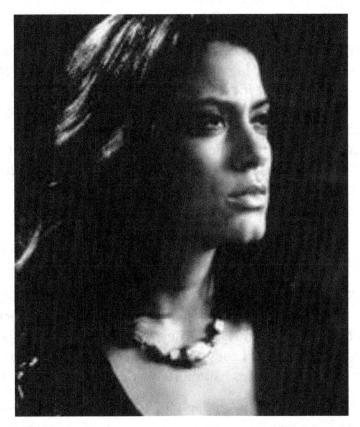

Status:
"The ultimate measure of a man is not where he stands in moments of comfort but where he stands at times of challenge and discovery." - Martin Luther King, Jr.
January 18, 2010

I have had many "one day my life was changed forever" experiences. I want to share one of those with you.

In 1971, my folks moved us to our first family home. I was six, my brother Charles Haasan was four and Fred was two. Haasan, Fred and I originally attended a daycare not far from the house. That wasn't a positive experience for my brother Haasan. There was very little one-on-one care for the toddlers (the rules were much more lax in those days). Haasan needed that kind of attention. He had many abandonment issues and would cry and throw tantrums for hours on end. I hated I couldn't take care of him.

My parents finally found a babysitter for us. I'll call them the Bads. They seemed like the perfect family. They lived walking distance from Bennett Elementary School, in a nice-sized lovely house. My memories are a little hazy about how many kids there were. I know there were at least two teenage girls, a preteen boy, and one boy my age. Mrs. Bad cared for Haasan and Fred during the school day. I went to Bennett for school and then would walk the short distance to their house afterwards. When the teenagers came home, Haasan and I were their responsibility. We would spend the day in the basement until our parents came to get us.

I loathed it.

Roaches OVERRAN the Bads' house. They were clean people for the most part but they were infested. There were so many roaches that they couldn't hide in the daylight. They were our constant companions. I spent as much time as I could in the stairway leading up to the first floor, since the other floors had more hiding places for the roaches.

There was a day I will never forget. Mrs. Bads needed some privacy upstairs so she brought Fred down to the basement for Haasan and me to watch. Fred loved to explore. He was so cute, shuffling around on his knees. I should have kept him up off that filthy floor, but at the time I loved to watch him go round in circles. When Mrs. Bads went upstairs, I put Fred on the floor and Haasan and I just laughed as we watched him speed around. At one point I noticed he had stopped. He was studying something on the floor with intensity. As I walked over to check it out, I saw the full-grown roach frozen in place by Fred's presence. I went to grab him up but Fred was too quick. He popped that roach right in his mouth and gobbled it down. Now I know that roaches are delicacies in some countries but I didn't know a thing about that at that time. It was just too much. I screamed and tried to get him to spit it out. It was too late. Fred just gurgled at me with a roach-eating grin on his face. Haasan immediately went and told Mrs. Bads. There was nothing to be done. She scowled at me and took Fred upstairs.

That event did not help me. I'm sure Mrs. Bad wasn't aware that leaving me in the basement with roaches was creating a phobia in me. I think she and the others were used to the pests. I was also taught not to complain or bother adults in any way. I just dealt with it. Later as an adult I was terrified of roaches but couldn't remember why. I had blocked out the roach phenomenon at the Bads' house. When I remembered the experience, I was able to let go of that fear. I still can't stand roaches, but now I understand why.

I also had to deal with three very human pests. The Bads teenagers did not like me for some reason. I can speculate why but I really don't have a clue. Maybe they picked up on the way I saw myself. They say, "If you don't love yourself, no one will." Well, I didn't. My negative self-image was probably very evident and bullies tend to gravitate to that energy immediately. I never looked people in the eyes and always walked with slumped shoulders. I didn't hold my head erect. I felt unworthy.

There were several reasons I felt this way. Unconsciously, I was modeling the behavior of my mother. She had very little self-esteem. Mom was extremely shy and constantly belittling herself, commenting about her weaknesses. I never witnessed her standing up for herself in any way. When people mistreated her (which was constantly — calling her crippled or fat or nigger lover), she would just put her head down and say nothing. I know now that she was "turning the other cheek" but all I picked up was that was the way to carry yourself. The crazy thing was that my mother was gorgeous. She did not see it. She saw a frumpy, overweight cripple. Our self-perception can be so skewed.

My opinion certainly was. Some of my feelings were also due to an emotionally abusive adult in my life. She was talented at hurting any and all people who allowed her to. Putting down weaker people strengthened her. Children were no exception. My mother didn't defend me early on; it just wasn't her way. She believed her love protected me and that was all I needed. Well, it mattered to me. I believed that woman, and I still fight that image of myself to this day.

The Bads girls sensed my hatred of myself. They were quite cruel to me. I blamed myself and didn't tell a soul. They began to abuse me. First verbally: They told me how hideous I was; rubbed in the fact that I didn't fit in. I was an ugly, yellow half-breed and nobody would ever be my friend. In those days there weren't too many children of interracial couples. Very few people looked like my brothers and me. For some reason, being a girl made being different worse.

Next the Bads girls moved on to physical abuse. They were very smart about it. One of their favorite ways to hurt me was at the park. They'd put me (all 45 lbs. of me) on the seesaw, lift me up high with their weight, and then jump off. I would slam down hard onto the dirt ground. I stayed sore. It was pretty miraculous that I never broke anything. They pinched and prodded me while they laughed mercilessly. Somehow they always managed to explain away my "boo-boos" as something I did to myself, even blaming my brother for some of my injuries. After a while, they realized I wasn't going to tell on them so things got worse.

Fred was out with Mr. and Mrs. Bads. Haasan and I were in the basement, enjoying afterschool cartoons on an old black and white TV. The house was unusually quiet. Eventually, the teens came downstairs. They carried a large, old, brown blanket and a brown paper bag. The preteen boy took Haasan upstairs while the girls beckoned me to the large dining room table. I was curious but also aware that something was wrong. They were rarely nice to me and they were smiling. I wanted their approval so much that I did what they asked. They told me to climb on the table. They wanted to play a game. After covering me completely with the blanket then sticking their heads in, one of the girls brought out a flashlight. The other girl brought out a large spoon. That is when the sexual abuse began.

Those girls stuck all kinds of things in me. That was not where it ended. They continued their horrible experiments with their own little brother. The teen brother brought their little brother downstairs at the sister's request. They then proceeded to fondle him to arouse him. They would then try to join the two of us. The boy always lost his erection though. He was never able to penetrate me. This went on several times over a year.

I knew what was going on was wrong but I didn't tell. I kept it all to myself. I didn't believe anyone would believe my innocence. I had already heard in church that sexuality was wrong if you weren't married. If you "messed around" in any way you were a sinner and God didn't accept sinners into his Kingdom. I didn't want my parents knowing I was going to Hell.

Thankfully the sexual abuse finally ended. I guess they got bored with it. Unfortunately, the new role of victim was instilled into my being for far too long. My brothers and I stopped going to the Bads soon after. I was very relieved but confused because I still wished for their approval when we saw them as we walked through the neighborhood. It never came. It bothers me to think what might have happened to those kids to make them do such horrendous things. Would their cruelty pass on to their own children? I hope not. I don't believe I'm going to Hell. I don't believe they are either.

Status:
"You say I am your fantasy, when all I want to be is your reality."
April 9, 2014

You Say

You say I'm your fantasy
When all I want to be is your reality

Business comes and business goes
But will you have remembered me?

You say you love me
When all I want is for you to show me
Hard times come and hard times go
But will you have remembered me?

You say I'm the only one
When all I want to be is someone
Frustration comes and frustration goes
But will you have remembered me?

You say we are forever
When all I want is right now
Disappointments come and disappointments go
But will you have remembered me?

No more emails
No more phone calls
No more voice mails
No more texts
No more Facebook
No more snail mail
No more pleading
No more begging
No more crying
No more. ...Nothing
But will you have remembered me?
I don't think so

Status:
"I am hopeful for positive change."
December 19, 2012

Sometimes I have to fight my genetic demons. Genes pass down our body types, hair and eye color, and medical history, but they can also pass down positive and negative personality traits. I have fought depression my entire life - I got it naturally. I wrote this one long, hard night a few years ago:

I woke up in the middle of the night with these thoughts again: Thoughts of suicide. I've often wanted to end it all, I'll admit. I am not afraid of death. The peace of it is constantly on my mind. But my daughter keeps me here in this place. I would not want her to have a loss as great as that: her selfish, weak mamma got tired and killed herself. That's not a pattern I'd like to begin. But still I ponder. I know there are others who could probably give her an amazing childhood. But to lose a mother like that at her age, at any age, would be devastating. And not fair. So if I died naturally or in some accident she'd be cool - but not the other way. So, I'll just go on.

I remember when I was a teenager my mother seemed to want to end it all. She spent many evenings and nights in bed, mourning. My parents decided to divorce after 20 something years of fighting and lack of communication. They had some good times but I guess not enough. Daddy finally moved us to Indiana and began his life anew in Chicago; without us. Daddy was the only man my mother really knew. She still loved him; he was gone, so she believed all was lost. Her primary goal was to make sure we (my four siblings and I) were fed, clothed and healthy (thank God Daddy paid most of the bills so we were able to survive). My mother would drag herself out of bed in the early morning to go to work. That was her only venture out of the bedroom. All the cooking (if we weren't eating fast food), cleaning, disciplining was now left to me. I was very sad about this. More than anything, I wanted to see my mother smile again; to sing as she washed the dishes, making chores a game as we spent Saturdays vacuuming, dusting and scrubbing the floors. Those days were over. Unfortunately, my little baby sisters never met the woman my mother used to be. So I just tried to take over for her. I tried to fill in for both my parents.

That's why I won't allow myself to just lie in this bed. I refuse to show my child the helplessness I feel. I don't want to continue this pattern of depression that runs so deeply within me. I have to hope for positive change within. Of course my daughter is very insightful. She can very often recognize the pain I hide inside. When she asks questions, I am very honest with her. I don't give her details that might bring her down, but I don't underestimate her ability to understand the state of things. And she often helps me. I don't want her to take on the problems of an adult. She deserves to have a childhood; but if I'm honest about my feelings, she hugs me and lets me know through her loving embrace that I am not alone.

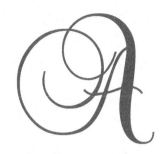

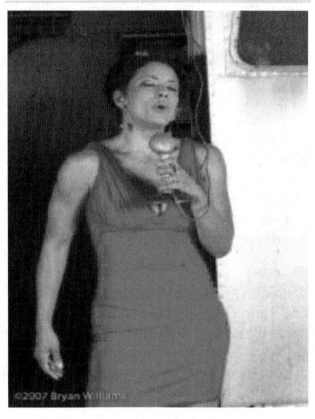

Ability

©2007 Bryan Williams

Status:
I'm singing again
December 9, 2013

I'm singing again. I thought it was too late for me. The music industry is so youth oriented, and I'm no youth, so I'd given up that dream. I never stopped singing for fun and a little cash (movie soundtracks), but to actually record a CD and perform live professionally? Yeah right.

Fortunately, since I sang "Harlem Blues" in my first film "Mo' Better Blues" my fan base has consistently requested more. I get comments like, "You can act but WHEN are you going to sing, again? Girl, what are

43

you waiting for?" That song is a favorite for a lot of people, which amazes me. When I sang it I had no idea what I was doing. The Jazz genre was new for me. But the lyrics... Oh, the lyrics... I connected with. I've always considered myself a storyteller and when a song relates a full life of experience, I can find a way to make the people feel it. I guess this is how my acting ability comes into play. When I met and performed with Branford Marsalis - Wow! What an experience:

I was scared to death to sing. I've sung in front of many people, but they were normal church folks or the community theater crowd. They always rooted for me. Sometimes there were sneers because I do have a different vocal quality than most; I can't do all the vocal runs you hear in the Gospel world. But ultimately, the audiences supported me with all my differences. I was in a special world now, the land of the professional musician. I was embarrassed at times because I am no expert at reading music and don't know how to play an instrument. I always wanted to learn but lessons and instruments cost money my parents couldn't afford. Singing was free.

Spike Lee made me very paranoid; he was such a Jazz aficionado. His dad was a great Jazz musician and they both were very concerned that I do a good job with this song. It was a major turning point in the film. It was the point that Bleek realized that his life as a professional trumpet player was over. I'd done enough plays to understand how crucial the climax of a story was. I never knew I'd play so important a role in my first movie.

For a couple of months, I'd been talking to Spike on the phone about the history of Jazz. He quizzed me all the time. I'd taken a crash course in the history of Jazz. It was all so much; and added to the pressure of learning this song and doing it justice. Thank God, Raymond Jones knew exactly what he wanted. He was pleasant, helpful and patient. He didn't have to be. Not everyone I had experienced to that point had been.

I'd never been in a real recording studio before. It was the day the orchestra was going to lay down the song. The strings warm up and I felt soothed by the sound. I was going to be all right. I was singing with them so they would have a basic idea how I would be laying down the vocals. My voice was in their headphones; scary. I hoped I wouldn't crack. But it was so exciting. The musicians warmed up as I settled into my soundproofed room. Then they began and I felt as if I am lifted away into the clouds. It was euphoric. These men and women were amazing. How blessed I was to be in this room.

For years I'd been very confused about what to sing. My beginnings were in the church, of course. I sang in the Jubilee Joy Choir in Muncie, Indiana. That was a wonderfully moving and inspirational education, but I've never had a traditional Gospel sound. I sang in many musicals, in alternative rock bands and I was classically trained for seven years. The joke in my family is that I am a black-a-billy. My Dad still believes I should sing Country - I love the lyrics of Country. Maybe with Michael Martin Band I can do some Folk. That's close enough to Country. But because of that first song, it has been expected that I sing Jazz. No matter that I never sang or even studied Jazz before I did "Mo' Better Blues" I thought the music was melancholy and I didn't need any superfluous causes for depression, but that's what the people want. Twenty years ago, I was not ready to commit to the style, but I believe I could now. Once in a while. What I will record first, I do not know.

Status:
It's been a rough week but I have remained productive. Thank God. Time for a little nap before I get up and out there again.
March 21, 2014

Choose to Write

When I am filled with sadness
When I can't see the light
When all my hope has vanished
That's when I choose to write

When there's nothing left to dream for
No potential within sight
When my spirit heart is broken
That's when I choose to write

When the darkness is relentless
When my smile has lost the fight
When my tears won't stop their falling
That's when I choose to write

When self-pity is my hero
And I'm in unending night
When my strength is forgotten
That's when I choose to write

When I want to stop living
Besieged by my plight
When death seems my only option
That's when I choose to write

When I choose to write
I can see through to the light
When I choose to write

Status:
"Are you acting, right now?"
December 5, 2012

Very often in everyday situations, people ask me, "Are you acting right now?"

Huh? I have been blessed with a gift for creating characters. I think it stems from the fact that I've spent so much time talking to myself and answering myself aloud. Yes, even speaking for the imaginary person in my mind. It is a self-therapy technique I created when I was very young. It made me feel better about any situation if I could just talk it out. I often wasn't brave enough to communicate to the actual person but I certainly could get into some imaginary confrontations - positive or negative. This naturally translated to building characters from the ground up. I love doing it and definitely want to do more.

But NO. Today, when I am communicating with a person as Cindy or Cynda, I say what's on my mind; right here, right now. That is because I am the worst liar on Earth. That's why I don't even try. When I am angry, I can't hide it. When I am pleased, the joy is written across my face. Every emotion is spelled out. Needless to say, I have never been a successful Poker player! Instead, I make it a point to just say what's on my mind, but I didn't always. I kept my mouth shut about my challenges when I was young; never telling my parents, any family or friends the things I was going through. I believe that made me sick.

When I was a young student at Ball State University, the acts of talking to myself and truth telling collided in the most embarrassing way. I was living in the campus dorms. I have many siblings (there are seven of us) so I was used to a house full of people (at the time six of us, including my mother, were crammed into a small three-bedroom house). But because I was the only girl in my family for years, I was used to having my own room. My little sisters didn't come along until I was 14 years old, so moving into a small dorm room with a stranger was a challenge. I am very clean and neat; probably because I've had so much internal chaos in my being, I've needed to control my surroundings to stay sane.

Of course, my roomie was the opposite. She was simply a slob. She could have cared less about the cleanliness of her body or surroundings. She carried herself as if she owned the world and it was her own private dumping ground, throwing her things (dirty clothes included) everywhere. She was a nice girl but knew nothing of boundaries. More than once I would come home to find some stranger she'd invited in my bed, my drawers opened, and my make-up, jewelry and clothes strewn about. As you can imagine, that did not go over well, but my natural inclination at that time in my life (not earlier when I fought on a daily basis but kept my mouth shut) was to avoid confrontation like the plague. I would just come into the room, smile and clean up my things. She would always apologize and I would accept, until one balmy spring night near the end of our tenure together.

I should mention I was an asthmatic. Every spring, summer, and fall brought me severe asthma attacks, induced by air pollutants and stress. The ONLY thing that controlled my attacks was the fan. I slept with my fan. The cool breeze gave a feeling of constant airflow to my lungs. That night I came home and my fan was gone! I knew my roomie had to have loaned it out or broken it... something. It was late. I was tired and PISSED. She lay sleeping soundly in her bed. I was too man-nered to wake her. What was wrong with me?! Instead, I began my nightly ritual of preparation for the next day. I got my little ironing board and iron out of my closet and began to press my clothes in the dark. I railed against her in my mind. "What a b! Messing with my stuff! I can't stand that fat slob! Always in my drawers, eating up all my food, smelling up the place! I wish she'd just go! I hate her!!!!!" Once I finished ironing my clothes, I gathered my things for a shower and left the room. The communal bathroom was right across the way. As I was washing my face, I heard a loud slam. I went out to see what all the noise was about. My fan sat in the middle of the doorway. My roomie was no-where to be found. I have to admit I was confused but happy. Maybe I could actually get some sleep that night.

The next day I came home for lunch. I rarely entered my room during the day. Why I did on this occasion, I have no idea. My roomie was pack-ing her things. When she saw me, she began to throw her clothes into her bag viciously. I asked her, "What is wrong with you and where are you going?"

She stopped and stared daggers into me, "Don't even pretend with me. YOU know, I KNOW I'm a slob. I'm sorry about that. But for you to talk about my eating disorder and weight is bull crap! You are a mean per-son, Cindy Williams. I refuse to live with you another minute."

I couldn't believe it. I had NO IDEA I was speaking out loud! I felt so bad. I never meant to hurt her. I didn't care about her weight. I was having weight issues myself. I just spoke out loud, the rage I had stuffed inside for so long. I momentarily forgot about the year of hell I'd tolerated with her. I apologized profusely and left her to it. How could I be so awful? I'm not a good person. God forgive me.

But that night I slept peacefully in my clean, pleasant-smelling, quiet solo space. Good riddance!

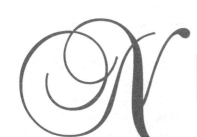

PINK PANTIE
CONFESSIONS

Naked

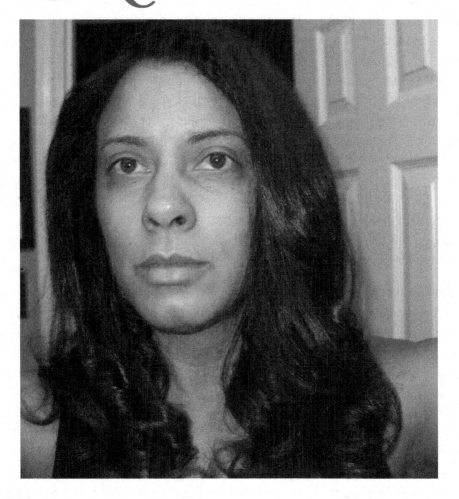

Status:
Success is not final, failure is not fatal: it is the courage to continue that counts. – Winston Churchill
July 26, 2013

I wrote this back in my audition days, thinking it was funny. It was also typical of my experiences while in L.A. You could say I was a little bitter when I wrote this. Yes, even this goody-two-shoe has those brief moments of bitterness. They fade quickly. And, like I said, whatever I am feeling at the moment, I'm going to write about or say out loud:

I was at another TV audition. It was for this new series PRIVATE PRACTICE. I really didn't like auditions. I have never been very good at this part of my career. There is so much more to it than acting...You have to walk into the room as the character. They say they want to meet the "real" you, but that's BULLCRAP. They don't care if you can act. They want a ready-made character. For instance, if the role is for a prostitute, you better have a great idea about what type - high-class call girl or street hooker - and walk in that room being her. When you introduce yourself, BE her. If she uses Ebonics in the script you better find it within yourself to speak it as if you grew up in da hood and never paid attention in Language Arts. "Hi. What's up chaw?!!! I'm Cynda Williams, niggah! Get it right! Can we do dis? I got thangs to do." It seemed like productions rarely expected actors to be able to act anymore. Was the art gone? I felt like I was surrounded by accountants with no vision calling themselves visionaries.

Another issue I had with this entire process - what I hated about it - is all the women piled into the room. There are SO many. Everybody was there to play opposite Taye Diggs. Did the studio even know what they were looking for? There was every conceivable sort of woman in that tiny room. Dark, light, short, tall, thick, thin... everybody and their mamma was up in that place! There were even Latinos and Asian chicks. Some were audition room friends. They'd go up for the same shows all the time, chatting mercilessly as if they weren't at all concerned about the job... but I knew they were. The way they would cut their eyes as someone entered the casting room; the way they would laugh shrilly at some stupid off-handed comment, distracting the rest of us who sat and tried to study. Then there were those who were just plain nasty. If you looked at them the wrong way and you might get your head cut off!

How tall was Taye? I wanted to know. He looked short on TV. He was a fine brother, but a little one. Dang...

I looked at a girl across from me. She was gorgeous, with long hair to her lower back, beautiful cocoa skin and she couldn't have been more than five foot four; if that. She might have weighed 110. I hadn't been consistently less than 140 pounds since I started college, eons ago. I hated my body and I despised coming to these auditions and remembering how unattractive I...There was another perfect girl with a 5'5" athletic build that, I was sure, stopped traffic. She had a short and slick bob. Her skin was flawless and chocolate. Darker women did more TV. They got the bulk of the doctor and lawyer roles; played the mothers and judges. The light-skinned women were the temptresses and hookers. This character was a doctor with her own practice. I didn't have a chance. Sometimes I hated being me. I wished I could be her... or her... or her.

I went into the room and what happened? The first thing they asked was, "How tall are you?" I hesitantly lied, "Five six and a half?" The casting directors decided that that was a good time to eat lunch and make a couple of calls. They let me audition, but I could read their body language; it said, "Hurry up, What-chor-name. I've got more important things to do!" I tried to reel them back in by giving a stellar performance with the hired audition actress, but they were gone. I said a brief "thank you" to the crowns of their heads and left. Another failure. When was I going to have some S-U-C-C E S-S?

Sad, huh? That is how I felt at the time. By then I had done quite a few movies and I still didn't think I was good enough. Acting is a tough business on folks. You get rejected far more often than you get hired. I had to learn to never give up. Thank goodness, MOST of the time, I could see through my self-doubt and understand that what was mine would come to me. I would get the jobs that were meant for me. The ones I didn't get, I learned to let go of. Only then could I have any peace and be ready to try, try again. I then celebrated the women who had been chosen. It was usually Halle Berry and Angela Bassett, etc. Those awesome women deserved every job they booked. They were selected at the right time for their journey. By the way, I absolutely loved Audra McDonald in the role for the Taye Diggs gig. She was PERFECT.

Status:
"Ground Yourself With Touch" – Tracey O'Connor – "
I Like This
March 6, 2014

Touch

Touching me
Me touching you
Your hands intertwined
With mine
Slightly moist because that's how you make me feel
Sublime
Feeling your slow ... strong ... pulse
As you envelop your sinewy arms
About my waist
Pressing my face
Against your chest
Whiffing your spicy miasma
I say, "Yes"
Your kisses skip lightly across my neck
Making my heart stumble   stop   start
Commune
A jolt of electricity
Called devotion
I swooooooooon
You save me from lonesome despair
As you gently run your fingers through my hair
Breathing in the warmth of you
If only you knew
How I miss you
When you go away
Yet another day

You are ... so far ...   away ...   away...

Status:
"Do not spoil what you have by desiring what you have not;
remember that what you now have was once among the things you only
hoped for." — Epicurus
April 21, 2014

Oftentimes life gets SO scary. Being an actress who works SOMETIMES has tested my faith on numerous occasions. I have had many days when I had no idea how I was going to pay my bills, had no clue if I'd ever work again. I think even the most successful actors have these fears.

A few years ago, 2008 to be exact, I was living with my brother while my husband was starting a new job in Chicago. I had been on tour with an exciting new play that collapsed because of the Great Recession. My daughter was going to school in Texas so I decided to let her finish the year before moving to Chicago with my husband. We had already been moving around a lot and I knew she loved being with my brother and his family so I stayed. It was a dark and scary time. You see that play was going to change my life. I was finally going to clear up my debt and buy that house. I wrote this passage in the middle of one long and lonely night:

This night is really testing my optimism. Here I am again, lying in this foreign bed, sweating, and so afraid. Sophia is snoring peacefully next to me. I envy her; her sleep is rarely interrupted. My brother's guest bedroom is very nice: Burgundy accents on the linens and furniture. I love it; for visiting though I've tried to make it our own. Sophia's happy, hopeful artwork adorns the walls. But these walls are not mine. It's crazy I feel this way. My family has made me feel VERY welcome. They love having us here. But we cannot be here forever.

53

I can't help but fantasize. If this room were Sophia's, it would be decorated turquoise with light blue skies and beautiful cumulus clouds. She would be sleeping with her favorite stuffed bunny in a canopy bed with flimsy sheer curtains closed around her. There may even be a mural of a horse on the wall; Sophia loves horses. The carpet would be plush blue, turquoise, and purple with a beanbag in the corner. Sometimes I'd sit there and watch her sleep. Not tonight. I'd be in my own sage green bedroom surrounded by feather down pillows, spooning my husband in my king-sized four-poster. I'd breathe in his manly scent and fall back into a serene sleep.

Nice fantasy. Back to reality.

My worries are often about money. Trivial, I know. So many people have nowhere to lay their head, no food to feed their children; death and sickness surround them. But I worry nonetheless. I have only a little debt but a little can be overwhelming when you're unemployed, have no savings and are unsure of your financial future. Before Sophia, I never really cared. I would gladly survive on peanut butter and jelly, but I am no longer a starving artist with responsibilities to no one but myself. Now I have the love of my life lying next to me. She needs clothes (she's growing like a weed), food (she eats like a horse), and a physical. For the first time in my adult life, I have to consider getting a job that is not entertainment related. What can I do? I have no real skills beyond acting and singing. I need money now. My husband is struggling also. Fortunately, he has a job, but I need to be helping out. I'm not used to not having my own money. Anyway, one job is not enough.

I'm considering getting a job as a maid. My family laughs at me when I say this. "How can you go from having a pretty successful career in movies as an actress to cleaning houses?" No cash flow and a screwed-up economy, that's how. No work for black women in television or movies unless they are super low budget. Who can eat on that little bit of money? It's funny. I've always loved cleaning houses. I like things to have order... to smell fresh. I've cleaned for my family, for friends, for free. Maybe that's what I'll do.

I didn't become a maid, but I would have if the situation called for it. The cleaning service is a noble profession.

I eventually got my mind together and did what I so often preach to others. I concentrated on my blessings. I was safe, fed, and surrounded by love. My child, whom I dreamed about having for years, was and is the personification of love for me. No career or money could ever be as important. My family was wonderful. We all had our health. Things worked out. They usually do. We still struggle. I think everyone does in some way or another. Life is a school. No struggle, no growth. God is Good. All the time.

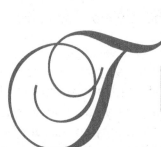

PINK PANTIE
CONFESSIONS

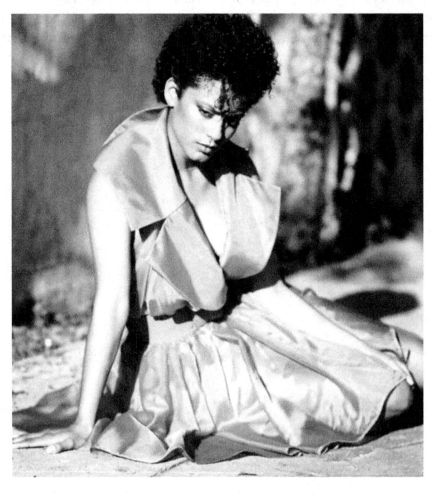

Temporary

Status:
"Temporary"
February 4, 2014

Where Black Is Brown is among many exhibits held at MAAA for its celebratory 40th anniversary year.

Did you know that 26 of the 44 founders of Los Angeles, called pobladores, were of African descent?

This photographic exhibition reveals lesser known facts about California & Mexican history.

This Event Is Free To The Public

The reception includes a drumming procession of African & Azteca dancers, musicians, dramatic performance, and a guided tour of the exhibition led by Curator, Toni-*Mokjaetji* Humber

Ethnic & Women's Studies Department

Cal Poly Pomona

A GROUNDBREAKING & BREATHTAKING EXHIBITION
SUNDAY, JUNE 5, THROUGH SUNDAY, SEPTEMBER 18, 2016
Opening Reception Sunday, June 5th 2:00 PM

WHERE BLACK IS BROWN

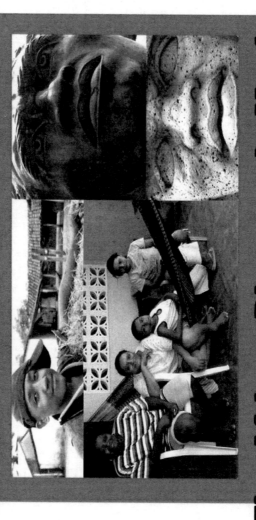

The African Diaspora in Mexico

The Museum of African American Art Los Angeles
4005 Crenshaw Blvd, Los Angeles, CA 90008 ∫ 323 294-7071
At The Baldwin Hills Crenshaw Plaza, Macy's 3rd Floor

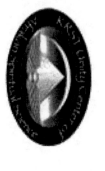

Krst Unity will honor Juneteenth with film screenings every Monday and Thursday evening in June from 6:00 pm to 9:00pm.

Films such as

Readings from Slave Narratives

The Cotton Picking Truth

And more will be featured.

Stay connected for complete lineup.

KRST Unity will commemorate Juneteenth each Sunday in June.

Portrayal of Slave Narratives—Sunday, June 5th

Slave Narratives Part II—Sunday, June 12th

Honoring Fathers and the Heroes of The Past—Sunday, June 19th

The Children's program "Building on the Wings of Maat"—Sunday June 26th

All commemorations will take place at the 10:30 am Empowerment Service

KRST Unity ALSO has a dynamic book study and workshop every Sunday morning at 9:00 a.m... It offers instruction on African-Consciousness from a spiritual point of view. Join Rev. Amadi Sadiki Hines as he explores the thoughts and teachings of several great scholars. The current book is Essays in ancient Egyptian studies Book by Jacob Carruthers BE SURE to stay for the 10:30 a.m. Empowerment Service.

KRST Unity Center of Afrakan Spiritual Science

7825 South Western Avenue, Los Angeles, CA 90047

323-759-7567 Office   323-779-9909 Fax

Website: www.krstunitycenter.org

Email: krstunityoutreach@gmail.com

"What you're going through? It's only temporary. Tomorrow's always another day." These were the most influential words my therapist ever told me. Every time I have moments of darkness, I hear those words in my head, "Temporary, temporary, temp..."

A good part of my yesterday was difficult. I was having "a moment." That's not unusual. We all face challenges. How I've learned to overcome my self-created barriers in order to progress makes the difference. There are times I find myself consumed with the unknowable future, overwhelmed with anxiety as I bellow in my mind, trapped in a circuitous monologue of what ifs? ... "What if it doesn't work out? What if I can't take care of myself? What if things never change? What if I never overcome my mistakes?"

Other times I become caught up in yesterday's misadventures; pulled into a dark hole of depression. Droning on in an inner whine of why dids? ... "Why did I do that? Why did that happen to me? Why did I deserve that? Why did they hurt me so?"

In the old days I would have ended up in a fetal position in my bed, under the cover of darkness, sweating with palpitations. Yesterday is daunting; tomorrow is ominous. Nowadays, I find a quiet place for about ten minutes and force myself to be in the now. "C, you have a home. This lack is temporary. You haven't known hunger for years. These troubles are temporary. Your body is healthy. These trials are temporary. Your daughter is happy. These obstacles are temporary. Your bills are paid. These difficulties are temporary. You have people who love you. This stress is temporary...You JUST got back from a dream vacation that was fully covered by the generosity of your phenomenal friends. These struggles are temporary!" If I truly see my life in the now, those what ifs and why dids dissipate safely into the universe where they can no longer cripple me, at least until the next time. I realize right now that all the challenges I've had, are having, and will have, are temporary.

This morning I awoke to another day: fresh and ready.

Status:
"One of the most difficult things about having a talent for understanding people is encountering those moments in time when you at long last begin to comprehend yourself. When you become aware of your own defects, you have to evolve...if you want to move forward. The metamorphosis hurts like Hell but that change can give you a peace/piece of Heaven."
February 18, 2014

I wrote this passage when I was being really hard on myself. I go through phases like that. I do not enjoy self-scrutiny, but if I find myself suffering incessantly over something or someone, I force myself to stop and figure out why. I'd venture to say the ache has nothing to do with outside forces. I am 100% of the problem. When I take the time to dissect my feelings, I naturally move on. I can't live in a state of blindness. When I finally figure ME out, the pain subsides.

I wrote these lyrics when I was feeling this way. The words indicate more drama than my story but theater makes for a better song. I even recorded it. For those purposes, it was a love song to someone else. I've changed a few lyrics to make it more a love song to me.

Ready For a Change

I've done so wrong; I've lived so hard
I've made mistakes so now I'm scarred
I thought I knew which way to go
But I was lost; now I know
I want a better life – I'm tired of pain and strife
Chorus
I'm ready for a change, ready for a change
My heart is not the same, heart is not the same
Eliminating shame, eliminating shame
    I'm ready for a change...
I hurt so bad, but it's all on me
Let myself down; my responsibilities
I'm ready for a change, live a brighter way
I want to be proud, starting today

I want a better life – I'm tired of pain and strife
Bridge: Not looking in the rear view mirror
It's time to move on, time to move on
I'm seeing truth so much clearer
It's time to move on, time to move on
Chorus

Status:
"Love Ain't Enough"
December 2, 2014

Quite a few years ago, in between husbands, I got involved with a man that changed my life. I'll call him Teddy (as in Teddy Bear). I'd met him while I was still fighting for my second marriage. He was a handsome guy to me. Beautiful smile, but not every woman would be attracted to him. At the time, he was very overweight, quite short; but I wasn't interested anyway. My heart was set on trying to rekindle the best relationship I had ever known. Nothing and no one was going to mess that up. Well, Teddy didn't mess it up. Time, water under the bridge, and changing paths did that.

After my husband and I split, I started going out to music, dance, and karaoke clubs. My cousin and I would get cute and go play. Dancing was our thing but we also went to hear Jazz, Spoken Word, whatever. We were single and ready to party; Los Angeles was awesome for that. Between the coastline, Mid-Wilshire, Leimert Park, the Valley, Beverly Hills, and Hollywood, there were vast choices of fun places to go. My goal was to find my way back to happiness. Teddy was a singer so we began seeing each other quite often. I'd go to a club and there he'd be on stage. He'd see me and smile, send me a drink, come down after the set and we'd just talk - talk about everything! And this man could make me laugh like I hadn't in a long time. I loved listening to his conspiracy theories - he was very paranoid - but the way he expressed himself was amazing. He was sometimes dark in his views. A people-watcher just like me, we could sit for hours guessing about the lives of the folks we viewed. The stories we came up with were very colorful.

You know it had to happen. We took the relationship from conversation to intimacy. That changed everything. I was falling in love with him. Deeply. He said all the things I wanted to hear and seemed to care about me. Though he cherished our time together he had a very independent life. A charismatic man's man, he had his own friends, own interests and left me to mine. He was a very talented, extremely smart man, and highly intuitive to my needs. Being the first to bring me out of my sexual shell, I thought I'd found my soulmate. But because I was barely divorced, I was not too keen on jumping into another relationship. I wanted to take it SLOW, to be done right. I'd had two failed relationships already.

The closer we got, the more possessive Teddy became. I was starting to have concerns but, alas, he was a magnet to me. I was head over heels in lust...I mean, love. Our relationship had a power that was palpable. It was too soon to commit but I couldn't help myself. The man moved me AND began to scare me. He started telling me about his past. He had lived a dangerous life. I wasn't sure if he was finished with that darkness.

Soon, his behavior began to frighten me. If I ever mentioned my desire to take our relationship slowly, he'd get viciously verbally combative. He threatened often that if I ever tried to leave him he would hunt me down. I believed him. But we'd had so many wonderful experiences together that I decided to ignore the red flags. I found myself, upon waking every morning, praying to God that Teddy would be nice to me that day.

Everything came to a head when one night I got brave and told Teddy that I thought we should not continue. We were at another club. He'd just finished his last set and was being especially mean. He was drinking too much and kept disappearing; leaving me alone with people I didn't know or trust. The energy was not right. "Please take me home," I implored him. He nodded his head then very gently veered me out of the club to his SUV. He quietly asked me to drive and I was relieved. Our phenomenal highs were being overrun with horrific lows. The cons out-weighed the pros. Never knowing if I would love this way again, I shuddered, but I felt danger and decided it was time to get out.

Driving home in the gloom there was a tangible silence. We were driving from Mid-Wilshire to my Valley apartment. It was after midnight on a weekday, so there was very little traffic. L.A. shuts down pretty early. We were making our way down Lankershim, just rounding the corner by Warner Brothers, when Teddy roughly reached over me, threw open the driver's door, and pushed me out of the car with all his might. He pushed me so hard I rolled across the street. Thankfully, there were no cars rounding that bend. As I lay in the street, breathing heavily, I saw him coming like a bull. His eyes were wild and he meant me gruesome harm: I saw it. I also knew he might have his gun. He always had it with him. I picked myself up and booked it across the street.

At that time, the L.A. subway was being built there. There was a stone wall separating the site from the street and I ran in that direction. Teddy caught up with me, grabbed me by the hair and began to slam my head against the wall. I fought back, screamed, kicked, bit - you name it, I did it. As I was beginning to lose consciousness, I heard a sweet sound: a young, male voice was yelling from across the street.

A security guard on his rounds had seen what was happening. He had a walkie-talkie and was calling for assistance. Teddy turned his rage onto the young man, yelling obscenities and making threats. The gun became forefront in my mind. I knew Teddy was going to the car to retrieve it.

Terrified for my naïve savior, I couldn't let the boy get hurt. "Teddy," I called, "Please leave him alone. I will never leave you. Promise. I will NEVER leave you. NOW let's go to your house and forget this ever happened."

Those words were the magic tranquilizer. He calmed and even smiled. We walked to the SUV, climbed in, and left. I'll never forget the young security guard as he shook his head at me in sorrow.

Teddy was crazy. That night I realized he was smoking cocaine all along. Now I understood his moods. A terrifying knowledge penetrated my mind. If I didn't get out, I was going to die. I knew it. He had insinuated that he had murdered before. Again, I believed him.

My sense of survival had now fully kicked in. I didn't want to bring my father and brothers into the equation to possibly harm or be harmed because of my rash decision to give my heart to a monster. I began a slow and methodical journey to freedom; I was determined to survive unharmed. Manipulating my way out of this, I began crashing the parties he had with his male friends. He hated me being around them. I stopped dressing up when I saw him, didn't brush my hair, teeth, or wash my face if I knew he was coming over. I allowed my apartment to look unkempt (and if you know me, you know how desperate I must have been to do that - I have OCD about neatness and cleanliness) and gradually began doing all the things I knew he despised. It was a slow process, but within three months Teddy let me go. He said, "I thought I knew you. You're just a lazy hoe." Then he walked out of my life.

I cried for months from grief and relief. I finally told my family so I would have a built-in deterrent for myself. I would never put my beloved male family members at risk of harm or prison time for murder. I cut the ties.

This abusive, sick man, I loved. Still do. Always will. BUT LOVE AIN'T ENOUGH.

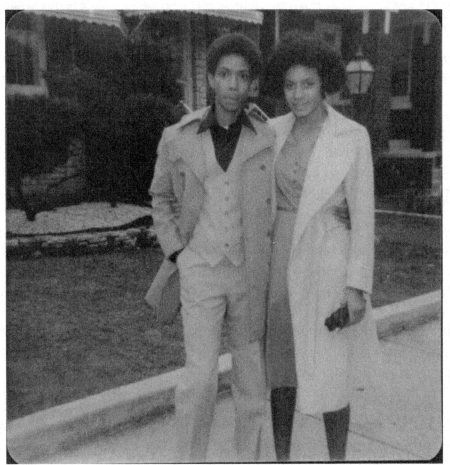

Carter Woodson and Cynda 8th Grade Graduation

Status:
"FIRST LOVE"
February 11, 2014

"Eros love – known as 'erotic love,' is based on strong romantic feel**ings towards another.** Philos love **- a love based on friendship between** two people who share a mutual, 'give-and take' relationship. Agape love - unconditional love that is always giving and impossible to take or be a taker. It devotes total commitment to seek your highest best no matter how anyone may respond. This form of love is totally selfless and does not change whether the love given is returned or not. This is the original and only true form of love." - David Nelmes

I found these definitions online attributed to Mr. Nelmes, but it was my grandfather, Rev. J.C. Williams, Sr. who, many years ago when I was a child, first taught me the concept of "different kinds of love."

Agape is what I strive for. It is how I know God loves me. When I became a new mother, I had physical pain within my gut when I held my daughter. The love was so overwhelming, I swooned with it. That may be the closest I will get to Agape love in my lifetime. Philos is a more prevalent type of love; it is the love of family, friends, and community. This select group has carved a place in my heart. Even when friendships with family members end, I will always love them. When I don't like my family, I love their dirty drawers... I may not stay around and smell them, but they live on in my memories. I'm a sucker for Eros. I love to be in romantic love. Who doesn't? This type of love is sometimes fleeting and often harrowing, but nothing compares to the feeling you have while you're basking in the rosy glow of the newness of it. I remember my first experience with Eros.

I grew up with boys - I adore them. I was the only girl in my generation for quite a few years, so my closest friends were male. I have a weakness for the smell of boys; earth and wind underneath sweat. I delight in their active and pushy energy. The boys in my family could never stay still and stay out of trouble. I would chuckle quietly into my hands when they'd be standing at attention while my father ranted on about their destructive behavior. I was affected greatly by the physical strength of my father. He would lift me high and twirl me in circles as I laughed uncontrollably. I truly believed he was a superhero. When Daddy spoke everyone listened. I love men who are strong in their beliefs and will speak on them (though I will admit I also need a man to respect and listen to me).

It's no surprise then, that I had crushes early on. My first crush was on a cousin. I was five-years old when my second cousin married a woman and adopted her son. I was completely taken by Bruce Lee at the time, so this Filipino boy who didn't speak my language thrilled me. Whenever I went to Ohio to visit my family he was my playmate. For about three summers I fantasized that he was my own private bodyguard fighting off dangerous intruders on the wild Chicago streets. He was my imaginary hero. As that crush faded, I set my eyes on a cutie-pie in fourth grade. This young man was a gymnast, so he was extremely agile and strong, and he had the most gorgeous smile. One day he sat next to me on the school bus after a field trip. Everyone was worn out from the day, so there was little noise. I was very shy and never said much. Seemingly out of nowhere, he quietly called my name and as I turned he chastely kissed me. I was shocked. Neither one of us ever said a word about it, but I will never forget.

The beginning of seventh grade was promising to be the start of an amazing year. This would be our first experience with multiple classes and teachers. I felt so grown. The prior year I had decided to change my life and make friends, so by now I had friends in every clique. I was extremely popular but did not like any one particular boy. It didn't help that my father made daily threats about my becoming involved with anyone. Like any father, he wanted me to "keep my legs closed and study."

The first day of school, my classmates and I were in for a surprise. A small group of new students had joined our school. These kids lived across the bridge; they had gone to another school that ended at sixth grade. I was overwhelmed with all the new faces, especially the one that sat across from me in homeroom. He was the most beautiful boy I had ever laid eyes on. He was painfully thin and wore glasses, but I liked that. I always had a thing for studious-looking guys. This boy had the prettiest redbone complexion and a copper fro! I had never seen an

African American kid with red hair. I must have embarrassed him because I stared openmouthed in his direction far too often. I even remember our impatient teacher threatening that she might move my seat if I couldn't pay attention to my work instead of my classmates. I knew who she was talking about. Carter Woodson. I even delighted in his name. I knew Black History very well and appreciated his parents for bestowing on him such a wonderful namesake.

Some time passed. Carter and I avoided each other for a while. He was as shy as I. But I remember when all that changed for us. Our homeroom teacher was droning on about some boring thing or another, when I felt pressure on my foot. I didn't move but my eyes shifted to his. Carter had a small smile playing at the corners of his thick lips.

I couldn't believe it. I moved my foot away. He found it again. It became a game that we played daily. Eventually we moved our affection from the feet to the hands when we walked home. We began getting to know each other as we headed to our separating paths. Carter was funny and smart, a winning combination for me (to this day, a man has to be able to make me laugh. I had had some difficulties as a child, so I was constantly looking for the pressure to be relieved with humor). He was gentle, yet strong. Opinionated, yet open-minded. And he listened to me. Carter became a support system that I didn't know I was lacking. I believe I was as good for him as he was for me. The first time we kissed, my little brother, Fred, caught us and threatened to tell my father if I didn't give him a nickel. That was the best nickel I ever spent. Carter and I spent the next 2 years being best friends. We had a very pure communion, especially because we didn't have past baggage to trudge through. Our innocent companionship fulfilled me.

When I had to move to Indiana in my ninth grade year, I was devastated. As young as I was, I truly believed I was in love. My heart was broken. I only went on one date a year (proms) from that point until I finally started seeing someone my senior year of high school. That's how long it took for me to move on.

My relationship with Carter became my template for partnerships. I've strayed many times from that template. I think I've had to have varying

experiences in my romantic life to grow as a woman. I've been strengthened, had joy, and learned to accept my partners as they are. I've made
mistakes, caused pain, and been wounded. It is an ongoing process.
Sometimes the pain has been so devastating that I wanted to give up
on ever feeling again. But I always go back to that first love and remember:

"Tis better to have love and lost than never to have loved at all." - Lord
Alfred Tennyson

Status:
I'm in love...with life and all in it...
October 30, 2011

In Love

I woke up thinking of your smile
You were living in my dreams
Reached over to touch you
Oh, that's right.
You're not there

The temptation is to moan
For your absence
Once again
But I won't tarnish my thoughts of you
By not loving life and all in it

I arose with your grin
Plastered on my face
The memory of how
You stroke your teeth
With your tongue
I laugh out loud
Loving life and all in it

I emerge into the light
I see flowers

Smell their perfume
I sing with birds
Increased by their glory
I breathe in air
Full and refreshing
I'm in love... with life and all in it
Because of you

Status:
I told my friend that breaking up leads to breaking down, but then you can break away, and BREAK OUT!
April 13, 2014

I have had my share of break ups. Some have been harder than others but they are all difficult. My normal behavior is to dive into almost every relationship thinking "forever." I have found that forever only lasts until it's over.

My cooper haired, scholarly FIRST LOVE and I shared some innocent times together. We had to keep our relationship a secret because I wasn't supposed to be "going with" boys at the time. I absolutely felt that First Love and I would last until the end of our time on Earth. Wrong. Life and circumstances beyond my control saw differently. Our break up was forced because I moved out of state. I have no idea where we might have ended up had that not happened. We were very close. I was extremely unhappy about the changes in my life so I grieved terribly when we said good-bye. My breakdown persisted for at least a year. I thought I'd never love again.

My dating was restricted to proms my first three years in high school. That was all my father would allow. He would scare possible suitors away by saying, "I don't want my daughter pregnant." This always offended me because I felt he didn't trust me. I had no intention of having physical relations with boys. I truly believed in abstinence until marriage. Daddy later told me he wasn't worried about my actions. He understood how hormonal boys could be. He didn't want me to be put in a precarious position. He said many innocent girls were assaulted by sexually hopped-up teens. I thought he was paranoid. I appreciated his protectiveness considering my painful past but I believed he overestimated the sexual prowess of these harmless Muncie boys.

I longed for a boyfriend. All the other girls had them by now. I was very shy but accessible, I thought. I tried to befriend the boys I was attracted to. They were cordial to me but they never asked me out. I thought it was my appearance. I was quite skinny. I had fair skin, unlike most of the other black kids. I was just an average student. I finally completely dove into acting, singing, and church. I essentially gave up. I tried to forget about my loneliness.

My senior year, I started to get to know a CHARISMATIC GUY that was extremely talented in theatre. Though not the cutest fellow, pudgy and dough faced, he made up for it with a wealth of skill. He was a well-rounded technician, actor, etc. I had admired him from afar for my previous three years in Muncie. We did a production of a well-known musical. I was fortunate to have landed a lead role. Charismatic Guy started walking me home after rehearsals.

Around the same time I met a very POPULAR junior. He was extremely cute and talented. He was playing another lead in the musical. I couldn't believe my luck when he and his brother invited me to lunch at Taco Bell. I'd NEVER had Mexican food before. LOL. At that time, McDonalds was the only fast food I'd had.

Two guys were actually courting me!

Charismatic Guy was a lot more aggressive. One day my father was in town and had his talk with him. He was the first to listen to my father fearlessly. Daddy's bulging red eyes and harsh tone did nothing to deter him from his advancements. Nodding his head he reassured my dad he had no intention of impregnating me.

After our show wrapped, Charismatic Guy informed me that he was having a cast party. We would be watching our show on VHS tape. When I showed up, we were the only people there. No parents. No other cast mates. No one. He showed me the film version of our show and proceeded to grab uninvited. He had no idea that prior to my time in

Muncie I was a street fighter so he wasn't expecting the slug across the jaw. I was very disappointed. My dad had been right. I had to be careful.

POPULAR became my first official boyfriend. He was the first to ask me out on a "date" date. I have to admit, I was afraid because he was white. To make matters more difficult, he was extremely cute with blondish brown hair and the prettiest cornflower blue eyes. Racial tensions were high in Muncie. I figured if I got my parents okay it would be fine. I was half white, wasn't I? My mother was mortified. We had a huge argument. I couldn't believe my white mother would deny me seeing a white man. She told me that interracial dating was painful and difficult. She was right but I didn't care. I liked him. Nobody else had the guts to ask me out. None of the black boys I'd liked for the last three years had ever given me a passing glance.

I stayed with Popular for quite a few years. We were good friends. We did experience crushing rejection from our peers but we had each other. I believed once again: Forever. I was wrong. We decided on a break my senior year in college although we stayed close. We dated other people but the plan was always to come back together.

By the time we moved to NYC the companionship came to an end. We wanted different things. Popular wanted fun. I wanted career and marriage. I wanted to wait for intercourse; he got tired of waiting. Who can blame him? I was an anomaly. He was so very patient. I've always appreciated the fact that he never pressured me. When we finally REALLY broke up, I thought all hope for long-term love was gone.

My next break up was pretty hard-core. It was another "love of my life." He was charming, gifted, intelligent, black as a BERRY, and gorgeous. My father actually liked this one right off the bat. Unfortunately, we both got it wrong. Let's just say Berry had no intention of waiting for marriage to get what he wanted. He just violently took my good stuff. I won't go into details on this one. Not here. Not now. We broke up. I broke down on every level. I questioned my good sense. I feared Hell. I was an overzealous Christian at the time – I made no room for terrible decisions and bad luck in my psyche. After much prayer, I eventually realized that God wouldn't deny me because a man I loved traumatized me. My virginity may have become a thing of the past but I still had a lot more living and loving to do.

My next guy was a JOY. He was very different for me. Joy was in no way connected to show business. Gorgeous, 5'2" and all man. He was a phenomenal chef and owner of restaurants. He treated me like a queen. I'm not sure if I've ever felt so safe and adored. I had many firsts with Joy. He took me to fancy places; we traveled together. I never had to worry about money. He spoiled me rotten. Joy took care of me and I took care of him emotionally. We NEVER fought. I was sure this was finally "the one." Nope. Of course we had an issue come up that was paramount. He wanted me to only work locally. Joy didn't like the thought of me traveling and working on location for films. He was very wealthy. I didn't need to work for money. He could take care of us until we grew into old age but I was IN LOVE with making movies. You have to travel if you want to do them. Was my love for him stronger than my love for my blossoming career? Before he asked me to make that commitment, I had already agreed to shoot a film on location. I decided to do the film and then come home to Joy for good... until I got there and could not give it up. I begged him to let me continue doing movies. He refused. We broke up while I was shooting a very difficult scene. He found a way to call me on set and demand my decision. I did. He burned my clothes. I only saw him one other time and he barely looked at me. Dreadful. I dreamt of him for many years. That was a major decision for me: Career over love. It broke my heart that I had to make it. I still sometimes wonder if I made the wrong move. I get tired of struggling.

My next connection was short, painful, and DAMAGING. THANK GOD we broke up. That's all on that for now.

My next relationship was lovely, for a long time. This handsome, competent, appealing writer was my BEST friend. He and I did everything together. Everything. Our time was fruitful. I've never felt so comfortable with anyone. We had very different lifestyles growing up but we just seemed to 'get' each other. I don't know why we broke up. Maybe we were too close. There was no autonomy. We depended on each other for everything. I still miss Best at times. He'll always be in my heart.

I had another bad one. See, "Love Ain't Enough."

Needless to say, I've been through numerous relationships and survived every break up. Every one of these journeys has taught me something new about the comings and goings of partnerships. They also taught me about myself. One: I don't give up on love. Two: I pick some crazy folks and some amazing. Three: I have many flaws. Four: I have much strength. Five: I'm still learning. I have yet to BREAK. I have grown from it all.

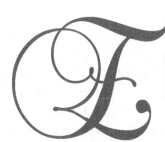

PINK PANTIE
CONFESSIONS

Evolve

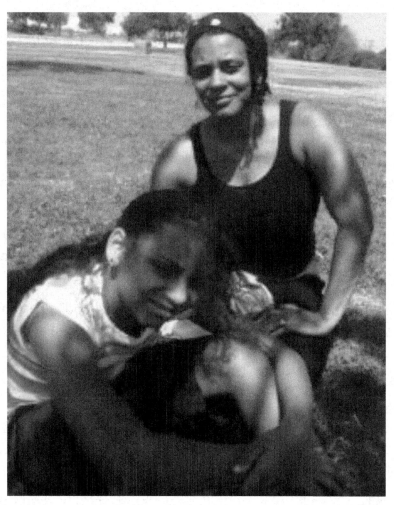

Status:
"Appreciation"
November 28, 2013

73

I was sitting at home in my bedroom alone watching the Sesame Street cast, The Roots and Jimmy Fallon perform "Somebody Come and Play" Thanksgiving Day 2013 in the Macy's Thanksgiving Parade. This was the first time I was not with my baby girl watching the parade on TV. She was with her cousins at my Dad's. I missed her so much. I realized sitting there (and not for the first time) how much this child of mine meant to me.

I wasn't always sure I wanted a child. Because I was the oldest girl of a large family and youth leader in my church, responsibility was heaped on me very early on. I thought I'd had my fill of that mess. I mean I missed out on having a normal teenage life! My existence consisted of going to church six days a week, school, singing and acting in plays, singing in the school and church choir, changing diapers, braiding hair, helping my siblings with homework, cleaning house, making dinner. I worked a few jobs. No parties, no movies with friends. Hardly had any friends for that matter.

There were times when I was bitter and couldn't see then how I was being taught to survive this difficult world. Learning how to make the wellbeing of others a priority, I was being made into a leader.

When I escaped to NYC I finally could play! I was a "good" girl so my idea of play was dancing and moderate drinking once in a while. I had fun. I'm glad I did it. Trusting only a few friends, I spent most of my time working and doing what I loved: singing and acting. I eventually moved to Hollywood and continued to have a busy life. I got married a couple of times; had moments of joy but to say I was happy? No. I can't honestly say I was. Part of the issue was I needed therapy and to cleanse. I eventually did those things but I still had a hole in my heart that needed to be filled.

Eventually, after a lot of living selfishly, I met my third husband and father of my child. Introducing Sophia Gabrielle! When she was born, the real "play" began. Sophia forced me to make a decision. Did I want to have a nanny bring up my child, or did I want to? Deciding to be a mommy meant I had to walk away from my career for a while. I won't lie. That, at times, was difficult but I wouldn't change a thing. My girl has brought a sense of peace to my soul. She filled me up in a way no movie ever could. Sophia, getting older is fiercely independent and very talented. Creating her own story, falling into her passions and bonding with friends means she won't be hanging around her mother too much longer. Cuddling my pillow alone on that morning was giving me a taste of what that would feel like. I had a deep appreciation for every moment I got to spend with her. That Thanksgiving I gave thanks to God for my daughter: The love of my life.

Status:
You know...Crazy things happen in life that you don't understand. How do you respond to the event? Will you be devastated into self-pity and/or stagnation? Or will you let this moment in time propel you to a renewed opportunity to trust the unknowable will of God? I choose the latter.
October 9, 2013

Loving Me

He smashed my heart and broke me down
Ain't got love for me.
His cruel words made me drown
Sadistic lies made me bleed
Vicious talk round and round
Cause I ain't loving me.

Loving me.
I've got to love me.
I've got to rearrange how I'm loving me.
It's me who's got to change how I'm loving me.
I'm loving me.

She loathed my body, soul, and style
Ain't got no love for me.
Filled my ears with bile

75

Her vicious lies made me bleed
My thoughts are mean and vile
Cause I ain't loving me.

Loving me.
I've got to love me.
I've got to rearrange how I'm loving me.
It's me who's got to change how I'm loving me.
I'm loving me.

Status:
"I'd rather be fruitful than busy. Working on knowing the difference."
October 30, 2012

I am very stubborn. Maybe that's the Taurus in me. I'd rather have something to blame it on. The stars...Yes, the stars made me do it! My husband used to tell me, "You work very hard but you don't work smart." Boy, would that piss me off. I thought he was being superior and condescending. When I was able to take my ego out of it, I realized he was telling the truth.

When I decide I want to do something, I work very hard to make it happen. It takes a lot for me to make a decision but when I do, I am rigid about making my needs and the requirements of others a reality.

My problem is, I rush in head first and start doing without thinking things through. I run with an emotional urging. I'm BUSY, BUSY, BUSY! "I'm going to help raise my nieces and nephews. I'm going to fix up my mother's house. I'm going to travel to my family and friends. They don't have to come to me. I'm going to be a mentor. I'm going to volunteer at the school. I'm going to clean my friend's house. I'm going to strip and paint my family's baseboards. I'm going to keep my neighborhood neat by picking up trash. I'm going to give my daughter the world." What the HECK?

I get so wrapped up in taking care of everybody that I lose myself. I still manage to cook, clean, write, go to all the games, teach, act and sing when I get the gigs, and pay the bills. I just exhaust myself so much from all the running and trying to satisfy everyone that I end up falling apart physically. Sometimes my brain takes a hiatus. I cannot think! I get sick and end up spending a week in bed.

As I grow more mature, I am finding that I need to be in a state of peace when I work. I am learning to slow down, breathe, and do only what I can. I can't do everything at once. Some things I don't accomplish at all. I'm discovering that if I don't do everything on my to-do list the world does not come crashing down. Sometimes, the best thing to do, is NOTHING!

I've succeeded at slowing my roll and found the results to be very satisfying. I have found I SHOULDN'T do everything. This is especially true when all my "doing" stops others from learning how to "do." I have to constantly remind myself that I could be taking a life lesson from my loved ones by doing it all. By arrogantly thinking I am the best person for every job, I unknowingly impede their blessings. For instance: I would love for my daughter to have everything her heart desires. She wants an iPhone, I'd love to get it; she wants to be in three sports, I want to make that happen; she wants a big house with a white picket fence, two dogs and three cats; sure...anything you want, baby! I have found that children don't benefit from being given EVERYTHING. Sometimes they need to learn to get it for themselves!

My daughter, Sophia, wanted a dog. The dogs we've had have not fit in our lives for one reason or another, so I got her fish. I can leave fish for a few days if I have to travel for work. So they're not cuddly and cute; at least my daughter has some sort of pet until our lives can support something more. I laughed when she realized, "Oh...I have to take care of my fish? I have to keep the tank clean? That can take at least an hour to do!" She was forced to be responsible for pets that take up much less time and effort than a dog. Sophia has learned from this experience. It was not meant for me to give her what she wasn't ready for.

Another example was Sophia wanted an iPad. Her dad and I didn't even have one! We couldn't afford to buy her an iPad. She wanted one so badly that she decided to raise the money herself. We told her if she raised half of the funds we'd provide the rest. She began doing extra chores for an allowance and asking for Christmas and birthday money instead of gifts. She saved for a year. Now Sophia has her own iPad that she earned. Her 10-year-old pride was immeasurable. If we had bought it, she wouldn't have learned the joy of self-sufficiency at such a young age.

In other words, sometimes the very work I need to do is to let others do for themselves. There is fruit in that effort. I am an old dog but I am still learning new tricks.

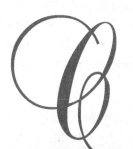

Called

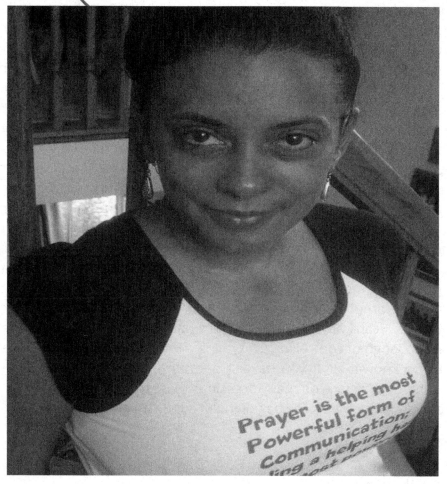

Status:
Pray that God will bring you the right people into your life.
April 15, 2012

Often times I post statements on Facebook that are meant for me. I tend to "preach most what I need to learn most." I believe in the power of making public statements of faith. I feel if I claim out loud in my private world and by the written word to a mass audience I might actually receive the blessings I ask for.

Many people come into our lives. A few are obviously awesome connections. I can usually tell if someone means me well. I can tell if they will benefit my life if only for a short while. Other times I meet a different kind. I have a very tuned-in BS meter. I'm not one to continue communicating with a person that feels wrong to me. The problem is sometimes the people I meet are what I need even if they are not what I want. They are sent to teach me something. No matter how hard I try to eliminate these people from my world, they stick like glue. The universe knows better. Maybe the person is a compulsive liar. I can't prove they are lying, but I just know. I can't stand that. I have no idea why they just won't go away. I don't call. They do. I'm not necessarily kind. They don't care. I can't bring myself to be a cantankerous jerk and send them packing, so they stay close. I have found people like this stay in my life for a season. When they do what the universe is leading them to do (even if they have no idea) they eventually pass on through and out like a dissipating foul smell; but I've been left cleansed. Before they leave, they tend to bring me some unexpected gift. I've met future employers this way. I've learned life-changing lessons of what not to do based on their mistakes. I can't always comprehend what's in the works for my life. I have to let go of controlling everything. That is hard for me. I can be a bit of a know-it-all, if you haven't noticed. I've had the harsh reality slammed in my face on many occasions that I truly don't know nuthin'. Understanding that is the beginning of a little bit of knowledge.

Status:
"Wake Up!"
April 30, 2014

Wake Up

Wake Up, Baby
I need to hear your voice

Your old mistress sleep
Has taken you away from me again
It drives me crazy how she demands all your time
I can't get a minute when she's nestled up inside your chest...
Rumbling deeply into your subconscious
Wake Up, Baby
Give me a little of that
The comfort she gives you is mine to give
How 'bout I give her the night so I can have the day
Or I'll give her the day
If I can have the night...I'd prefer it that way
I'm not selfish.
I can share.
I've even shared my bed with that mistress sleep...
Once in a while... when you're not in my mind...
BUT you've taken up residence there.
You rumble in my soul. She can't find her way to me
Wake Up, Baby

Status:
The Hater Blues
April 13, 2014

I follow politics. I can't help it. I have a very politically passionate family. We have our opinions, though I usually keep mine to myself. I believe people have the right to have faith in whatever ideology they choose. I try not to judge even if I don't agree.

I have some staunchly Republican friends and some deeply Democratic friends who ask me, "Do you think Barack Obama has changed a thing?" I always say a firm "yes." I do believe he is a part of a system that needs major rectification. He has disappointed many but he HAS changed things. His very presence in the office has transformed our conscious-ness. I won't go through his list of accomplishments nor will I recite his blunders. All you have to do is go to the Internet for that info. I tend to look at life from a different perspective. I contemplate events from a place of spirit. Barack Obama's presidency has shifted the mindset of our world.

For the first time in US history, someone other than a male from European descent is in charge. In spite of our dismay with the country's direction, the United States is a beacon of light to many. Others see the evolution of the planet's consciousness through our journey. For far too long the US has been a white man's world. Now there's nothing wrong with white men, I love them... but influence should not rest solely in their hands. It's time for forward movement. Many say we need to go back to the "good ole days." Those days weren't so good for anyone, including Caucasian men. You cannot consciously disparage others and not eventually reap what you sow. President Obama shows us that progression is eminent. A man of color can pilot this country effectively. A woman can lead. We've seen this in many other parts of the world. Women guide, other ethnicities show the way. Here too, even with our harsh history, we continue to navigate through. We can advance to include all.

This change has brought about hope. It has also brought out much hatred and fear. I have had to fight discouragement because of the intolerance I've witnessed. Writing these lyrics helped me.

The Hater Blues

(Melody of "Harlem Blues")

You can never change what's in a hater's mind
And if they feel entitled well there's no use even trying
Just like a mountain they are hard to move
Holding fast to the past and untruths, oh so fooled

The folks I loved, well they just turned me down because I am brown
Sometimes I feel such sorrow when I see them frown because I'm around
They stereotype me, as no other should, no, no

Then they surprised me, turning their back saying, "I'm no good."

And since Obama became POTUS
Hatred's reared its ugly face
Loathing, fear, animosity all over the place
I think I'll stand up for this land
I have nothing left to lose
Wanna drive off these mean ole Hater Blues

You can have your old ways, give me light and energy
I'm ready for a new day people, in this brand new century
From exclusion to inclusion, love and harmony
Ready for a revolution, now we're the majority

There are some spots in our country where I'm told its sudden death
To let somebody see you even stop to catch your breath
And if you've never felt the hate then I guess you'd never know
The chains of these mean ole Hater Blues

Ah, one day we will reach it; equality for all
All colors, genders, rich and poor, will come to heed the call
We are all in this together if we only choose to lose
The restraints of these mean ole Hater Blues

And since Obama became POTUS
Well it ain't the same ole place
Though a thousand liars smile right in my face
I'll think I'll stand up for this land
I have nothing left to lose
But the bonds of these mean ole Hater Blues

There are some spots in our country where I'm told it's sudden death
To let somebody see you even stop to catch your breath

And if you've never felt the hate then I guess you'd never know
The shackles of these mean ole Hater Blues

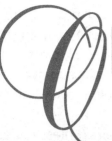

PINK PANTIE CONFESSIONS

Outcast

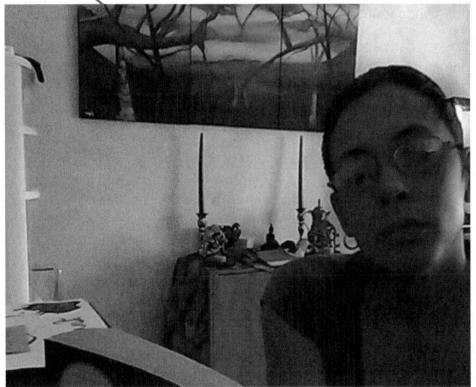

Status:
Confessions of a Nerd
February 24, 2014

I am a nerd. There's no doubt about it. I always wanted to be cool. But it just ain't happenin'. It took a lot for me to say that, because it bordered on cool. I am going to share with you my top 20 confessions of nerd-dom.

85

I am shy. I don't introduce myself to people. I wouldn't know what to say. When someone is sweet enough to approach me, I open up like a flower. Most people can't be bothered and assume I'm aloof. Being aloof insinuates being above it all. I am nowhere above anything. I'm just trying not to hyperventilate around all the newness. I'm articulate when someone comes to me with a "problem." Otherwise I have been known to trip over my words and I might find myself, mouth hanging open mid-sentence, forgetting my previous thoughts especially if I'm asked my résumé. Thus, I am terrible at industry affairs (unless I put on the "Cynda" outgoing actress persona).

I never had a good sense of fashion. I could care less about brand names and "who is wearing what." I grew up wearing hand-me-downs thanks to a generous friend in Muncie, IN who passed her used clothes to me. I was always a couple of years late with my attire, so I didn't care. That is why you'll find me in leggings and t-shirts if you pop in on me at home.

I organize my clothes by color. Some might call that OCD. I might agree. My closet goes from darks to whites. The winter clothes are to the left and the summer clothes to the right. The same goes for my drawers and shelves. I have managed to eliminate excess garments that I don't wear anymore so I can fit the entire wardrobe in half a closet. Most of these clothes are my audition costumes.

I don't wear make-up. Yes, I do wear it for gatherings and when I work, but that is all. I can't stand the feel of it on my skin. I do admit there are some wonderful products out there. I use MAC when working. It is very light on the skin. But when I'm just being Cindy, I want a clean face. Maybe when I age more that will change. Maybe that is why I haven't aged sooner.

I love to read - all the time. Books were my best friends growing up. I usually read 3 books at a time – a non-fiction, a spiritual text, and fiction. Don't be surprised if you see me reading children and youth novels. I love them all. Novels have saved me from curling up in a corner and giving up. I can always escape to someone else's world to be reminded that mine is pretty dang-on blessed...Dang-on...See...Nerd.

I don't curse really well. My friends in school used to try to make me mad just to hear me swear. See, I never heard bad language in my home. Never. My brother Haasan would test the boundaries and get his mouth washed out with soap. I had no desire to suck on Ivory with him. When I booked "Mo' Better Blues" Spike Lee gave me special lessons on how to be realistic when I swore at Bleek. He did a great job. My swearing ability soared after that but I still feel uncomfortable with it.

I love smart men. Every man I have ever had the pleasure of spending time with has been a genius in some way. Often book-smart but not always. Sometimes life smart. If a man can't teach me something, I'm not interested. Other women judge by looks, some by riches, some by fame. What I care most about is, "Tell me something I don't already know." And there's a lot I don't know!

I love to clean. When I was a child I had to help my mother take care of the house. She has always had physical challenges and could not handle keeping the housework up alone. My grandmothers were from the school of "you get every nook and cranny." When I clean it takes time. A lot of it. I do the base boards, wash the walls, clean the refrigerator, wipe the cabinets, scrub the floors, scour the toilets, wash the windows, vacuum the couches, etc. My home is spotless. I believe it comes down to keeping control of my surroundings.

My life has been unstable at times. I love acting but it is a very insecure vocation. You never know when you'll have to get up and go, if the money you make will be enough until the next gig, if you'll ever work again. There's nothing steady about it. If my home is organized and clean, my mind feels more at peace. I have had to learn to loosen up a bit with roommates and partners in the household, though. Not everyone has the same hang-ups as I.

I cherish school. I was an average student. Good grades did not come easyily to me. If I wanted to do well, I had to study. I had a natural knack for studying. I never was a crammer. I understood I needed to take in information gradually and consistently over the time it was presented in order to be able to absorb it all. I don't remember a class I didn't like.

87

I didn't understand math though. When I looked at numbers it felt like I was attempting to read a language I could not comprehend but I still loved being in the class TRYING to get it. I never did completely "Get it," but I managed B's most of the time (except that time in Algebra 2 – thank God for my teacher. He worked with me till I got my C. God bless him).

I am not the best dancer but I LOVE to dance. I was trained in Jazz, Modern, and Tap but that is not the same as Free-style. I will go to a dance club, go out onto an empty floor by myself, and boogie my butt off. There's always some smart-Alec who says, "You dance like a white girl." I just laugh and say, "I am half white." That whole thing of white folks not being able to dance is history though. Most of these hip-hop loving kids keep up with their Black, Latino, and Asian counterparts. I will dance until I drop.

I get excited about grammar. I love learning the proper way to write something, or say something. The other day on CBS Sunday Morning News a guy was talking about when to use "I" versus "me" in a sentence. I couldn't wait to share that info with whoever would listen. My daughter was the only interested party.

I am capable of changing my tone and lingo at the drop of a dime. I have a good ear and I listen. I understand that to communicate you have to speak the language (not foreign languages folks – although that is one of my few regrets in life: I wish I knew Spanish). Stick me down South, out East, in the hood, in the classroom, in the burbs, anywhere, and I can be understood. But I love to speak English in its pure form. I told you, I am a NERD.

My favorite channel is the Science Channel. Next is Animal Planet. Bio is a close third. I love movies about science especially natural disaster movies. I want to see what technology is used to solve the problems. I'll even watch The Sy-fy Channel for a good futuristic, end of the world narrative. The acting is sometimes under par and the plots can be predictable but I can't help but be pulled into the drama.

I always wanted to wear glasses when I was growing up. I adored the way other people looked in them, especially boys. I rationally know bad eyesight is not equal to intelligence but that studious look does something to me. Now that I HAVE to wear glasses, I'm not so keen on it for me. LOL...

I never smoked. I know these days smokers are losing their "cool" status but when I was growing up, you were a bore if you didn't smoke. All my actor friends would lean on poles with coffee in one hand and a cigarette in the other. They'd take bottomless inhalations and have the deepest looks in their hooded eyes like they knew all the answers in the world. I've always been allergic to so many things, including nicotine. I wasn't able to get in on their smoker's club. Boo hiss. But my lungs celebrate my nerdiness every day.

I was never a party girl. I prefer small groups to large. I feel claustrophobic when there is too much noise and too many bodies. I can't endure loud braying and being pushed. I think I may have gone to one party my entire four years of college. I only remember one. It was an actor's gathering. It was so crazy for me. I didn't do drugs, drink, or orgies so I did not fit into the scene at all. The only party thing I enjoyed was dancing, but those actors rarely did that. They had too many important things to say as they hovered around the party favors. I think my behavior at that party was the last straw for my boyfriend at the time. I was supposed to fit in. Do what they did. I didn't. He did. When I moved to LA I know I offended some folks. I would find a corner and read with the parties roaring around me. Who does that?! A nerd.

I love trees, plants and flowers. I am a nature girl through and through. Green is my favorite color. I love to be outside in it all.

I abhor litter. I have been known to stop in the middle of a sidewalk and pick up trash. I do not understand people who care so little for their homes and neighborhoods that they will throw garbage into it. One time I was with some new friends and we got some take-out. One of the guys threw his remains out of the window. I was flabbergasted. I felt hot and angry but couldn't say a word. I was afraid they might toss me out of the car if I said what I felt. My passion runs deep about keeping our Earth clean.

More on that: I recycle. I try not to waste anything. My daughter goes further than I. She makes artistic projects out of trash.

I say thank you and please.

I get angry if someone parks in handicap parking places. My mother is physically challenged so the nerve of a capable person taking those spots makes me want to fight. But because I'm a nerd, I don't.

I have many, many more nerdisms but I won't drone on. I just wanted to proclaim that I am a proud member of the Nerd Nation. Hear me...Whisper.

Status:
"I am a child of God. So are we all..."
December 18, 2014

Child of GOD

You think I'm ugly.
You think I'm weak.
You think I'm shallow.
A lowly freak.
You think I'm stupid.
You fear my skin.
You think I'm helpless;
And full of sin...
You don't know me!
I'm no different from you.
How can you hate me?
When God made me just like you?
Just like you.
You think I'm simple.
You think I'm slow.
You think I'm foolish

But you don't know.
You think I'm useless
Can't win the prize.
You think I'm dreadful
And so unwise.
You don't know me!
I'm no different from you.
How can you hate me?
God made me just like you.
Just like you.
He made me too.

Status:
"Actions Speak Louder Than Words"
January 12, 2014

I've never had a lot of friends. The few I have are phenomenal people. I'm attracted to out-going, light filled, gregarious men and women – people opposite from me. I have always been quiet, shy, and somewhat unsure of myself. I am a listener. I can be in a room and disappear. That is how I am able to create characters. I learn to "act" in a different persona from those I watch. I love for my friends to be the center of attention. They make me laugh and come out of myself. They are a gift to me.

Over the years and since therapy, I've learned to pretend I'm not shy. Once I've spent enough time with a small group (large groups overwhelm me unless I'm on a stage) I can convince myself that yes, I am funny and charming. I'm not a good liar though. If I don't feel right about someone, I will remove myself from their presence, but not always. A few times in my life I have liked a person so instantly, because of their brilliance, that I have forced myself into their lives. I crave that light but I have found that even the most beautiful people are not meant to be my friends. It doesn't matter how hard I try, there are those who don't like me. I don't know the reason. Maybe it's chemical, or spiritual. Maybe I look like someone harmful from their past. I never know. I probably never will. I had one specific experience that altered my perspective of relationships:

It is 12:38 a.m., two days before Christmas and I was tired; past exhausted, truth be told. I had been painting for hours. I agreed to paint a rec room for a friend; my girl. I thought. I was starting to realize our relationship was very strange. I had very few friends in Los Angeles. I'd never been an outgoing person and trusted very few but I loved this woman. She had always seemed like one of the nicest people I'd ever met. I would do anything for her and I had done a lot. I started recognizing the fact that we didn't do things as friends do. We didn't go to movies, talk on the phone, spend time together, talk; nothing. The only way we related was when she wanted me to do something for her. "Cindy can you come over and watch the kids?" Yes, of course. "Cindy can you come clean the house for me? I can't take care of the kids and clean. It's just too much." Sure; you know I will. "Cindy this house is so ugly. Do you think we could paint these rooms? It would be so fun!" Then I would get to work. We'd certainly talk, then, about what we were going to do next.

In the beginning she would help. She enjoyed learning how to do new things and had plenty of money to experiment. She'd buy every tool necessary, every book about the subject. No expense was spared. She never worked a regular job while I knew her, but her husband made sure she was taken care of.

But later, she started to get depressed. I wasn't sure why. Remember, we didn't talk. I never knew what was wrong with her. I felt helpless to make her feel better so I kept painting and scrubbing and anything else she asked. I loved her that much and I wanted to help.

Everything changed when she was pregnant with her fourth child. This pregnancy had been difficult and she'd been mean; almost wicked. She knew that I had very little self-esteem and valued her relationship too much for what I'd gotten in return. Just the ability to say I had a friend in this lonely town. And she was taking advantage of me...

She gave me two days to paint a room. The design she wanted was difficult and time consuming so I'd been pushing myself to the brink to get it done. I finally completed it. I started to clean up the mess then heard a loud gush. Water was coming from somewhere at a rapid pace. I dropped the brush and rushed into the kitchen. A pipe had burst and boiling hot water was spouting out of it. The water was too hot to reach unprotected so I couldn't turn it off. I didn't know how to cut the water line. I was an actress and some-time painter, not a plumber! I didn't know how.

I ran upstairs to my friend's charming bedroom where she is sleeping peacefully. It stopped me short, but then I remembered why I was here. I whispered urgently, "You need to wake up." She was a very sound sleeper so I would have to raise my voice. "I need to talk to you. It's important." She rolled over and hissed, "What do you want!? I'm trying to sleep!" I said, "There's a problem downstairs. A pipe has burst..." She cut me off, "Then get down there and TAKE CARE OF IT! What are you good for? Now, get out of my room and leave me alone!"

I couldn't believe it. Here I was spending my holidays working for a woman who could give a doo doo about me. She never was my friend. She'd charmed me. Smiled at me and made me feel that if only I'd do for her, she'd be my friend. Sure I was invited to the parties but I never quite fit into the scene. That wasn't her fault but this was unacceptable. How pathetic I'd become. My body started to quake with anger. I didn't know if I was angrier at her or myself. I had been able to control my temper for years but now I was afraid I might fall back into my violent scrapping days with this thin pregnant weak woman. I really felt like jumping across that room and ringing her neck. I wanted to shake her back and forth, up and down for all those years of subservience and degradation. I backed away a step and emotionless said, "Get up and take care of your own house. If you don't do something your entire first floor will flood within the half-hour. Good-bye." I walked back down stairs and made my way around the flood. I cleaned up the freshly painted room as best as I could; I wouldn't leave a mess. I then gathered my belongings and left by the back door. That was last time I ever did a thing for that woman without payment. I finally realized I was her un-paid servant; that was all. Our one-sided friendship was now over.

That was my fault. Totally. She was not a bad person. She was making the best of an awkward situation. I thrust myself into her life. She needed help and took it from a gullible person who was trying to make something out of nothing. I did learn a lot about house improvement. More importantly, I learned you cannot make someone love you that does not. "Actions speak louder than words." If a person doesn't act like a friend, they're not. I have to love myself enough to let go of situations like that. There are "many fish in the sea" with every relationship; part-ners, lovers, friends, sisters, brothers, etc. I deserve the best and so do you. Don't settle for less.

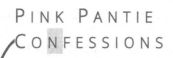

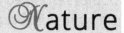

Nature

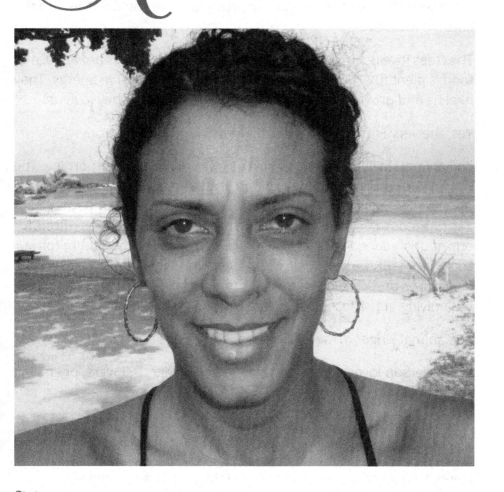

Status:
"I am thankful for all the love I have in my life"
November 28, 2014

I have love in my life. Always have. The world is full of love. We are pro-vided for, if only we'd notice.

The sun loves us. It feeds us nutrients, light and warmth. It loves us.

The waters love us. We are abundantly given "Adam's Ale" to keep our bodies refreshed and revitalized. It cools us and cleans us from the inside out. It loves us.

The atmosphere loves us. We are given invigorating oxygen to fill our lungs with life. It causes respiration. Without it we could not survive the Earth. It loves us.

The trees love us. They make sure the rains fall, shelter is provided, and food is plentiful. They cool us, clean our air, and conserve energy. They heal us and provide a habitat for our animal friends. They love us.

Yes, the very Earth itself loves us. When will we love it back?

The animals love us. The birds give us free concerts every morning. The worms turn our soil and make it rich for the crops we grow. Dogs, cats, horses, pigs, mice etc...allowed us to take them from their natural habitat to be our best friends. Numerous animals' lives are sacrificed for our nourishment. We rarely ask permission as we breed them for our sustenance. Butterflies fill us with glee as we watch their dance alerting us for days of spring. Spiders keep our insect sisters and brothers from multiplying at too fast a pace. They love us.

The animal kingdom loves us. When will we love them back?

Some person loves you, whether it is family, friends, lovers, or smiling strangers that cross your path. They love you.

When will we love them back?

Love (GOD) loves us. All above is not possible without her/him. You are loved. I am loved. I am thankful for all the love I have in my life.

Status:
Sitting in my family room with a steaming cup of joe, smelling incense, listening to the song of the birds through the window. Need to work out, write, and then get on with the work for the day but I want to savor this peaceful moment.

May 23, 2013

Fly Free

Early to rise I turn and sigh
The Cardinal sings then gives me wings
He brings reprieve
Helps me believe
I can flee
And be free
I soar along and sing his song
Does he hear me?
Sing in his key?
He gently glides and I'm in stride
This cadence always pleases me
His melody skips rhythmically
I want to wear his blood red cape
I'd disappear and escape
In my dreams, I fly free
The cardinal flies high with me

Status:
"Dear God, I start with a resounding, "THANK YOU!"I believe in your healing mercy. I know you perform miracles. THANK YOU for healing us of
the spirit of greed that runs rampant in our nation. THANK YOU for curing us of the lie called "lack;" the notion that "I refuse to share my blessings with those less fortunate because I do not have enough." THANK
YOU for alleviating us from the diseases of fear and hate. I declare all
these miracles because I know you can do ALL because YOU are the ALL
POWERFUL. I claim these gifts with total faith... of a mustard seed.
THANK YOU again."
March 20, 2014

I believe in a higher power. I was raised that way. If I had not been, I still
think I would be a believer. I have seen too many miracles. I've witnessed too many "coincidences" that were no such thing.

There have been times when I've seen Angels. When I was a teenager I witnessed an angel as it came to give my grandfather a message while he preached. My grandfather was very upset this Sunday. His assistant minister had, by then, betrayed him. This man he'd trusted had taken half of his congregation away to another church. To make matters worse it was the youth that he co-opted. My grandfather ranted and raved that day. He was going on and on. His tirade started to be unintelligible. This went on for at least an hour. I was worried for my Poppa. I had never seen him this out of control until... I felt a presence behind me. As I looked back over my right shoulder I saw a being shaped in the purest light. It stood as tall as the high ceiling of the church. My grandfather saw this at the same time I did. Poppa abruptly stopped speaking as the angel made its way to the pulpit. I noticed that the congregation had no idea what was happening. They looked around at each other in dismay. They understood the pain and embarrassment my grandfather was facing. Some of the men began to rise to assist him. My grandfather waved them away as he watched the angel come his way. As the angel reached my grandfather he looked up and listened. I couldn't hear what was said. My grandfather nodded his head saying, "Alright. I'm going to shut up now. Choir sing." I watched the angel dissipate in front of my eyes. Poppa sat down without another word. I was full of wonder.

I believe in Science. Science is the gift GOD gave us to understand his/her creation. I believe in evolution. Why can't it have been GOD that caused the big bang? Why couldn't GOD have created this world in his/her timelessness? Why couldn't he/she create the dinosaurs and other species we'll ever know about? Why must we put limits on GOD?

I believe there is evil. I have observed evil up close and personal. There are many beliefs about the nature of evil. We live with what some believe is "natural evil" every day. Some people focus on natural evil when they are trying to prove the lack of a GOD. "How can GOD exist when he allows earthquakes, floods, and famine?" I believe that the Earth has always replenished and rejuvenated itself. For the millions of years before our species was here, the Earth died some small deaths and some monumental, in order to evolve into a more wonderful place. Just because we conscious creatures are now here, we can't expect Mother Earth to stop moving and growing just to satisfy our desires.

There is material evil. Pain, disease, grief and sorrow plague us all. "How is there a GOD? He allowed my child to die. That baby was born with deformities. He allowed that murderer off the hook. Why didn't GOD strike Hitler down at birth? Why did this person betray me and get away with it?" I believe this Earth is a type of school for us. Things we don't understand happen all the time. We can't see everything. I believe GOD knows all. If I lost my child I know I'd question him/her harshly. I would be angry. I might even curse and want to die myself...but I'd still know there is a higher power.

There is moral evil. Murder and rape are daily occurrences. Greed runs rampant. A handful of people own a majority of the world's wealth. They are so gluttonous, many underpay and cheat their employees without a second thought. There is very little compassion for the underprivileged. Apathy is commonplace. People step over the homeless as if they are garbage littering the streets. Racism and prejudice are proudly touted by the ignorant because of fear. Human rights laws are willfully and with consciousness perpetrated against whole races of people while the world's religions turn their heads away with not an ounce of shame. People massacre in the name of GOD and call it righteousness.

We knowingly destroy our planet with no forward thought. None of these acts can be blamed on GOD. These are man-made decisions and acts.

There is supernatural evil. I believe this is energy that is the opposite of light. The universe has to have multiple layers for balance. In order for us to comprehend good we have to at times observe evil. I've had many experiences where I've seen it up close and personal.

When I was younger I saw beyond the visage of the "natural" all the time. I had not yet learned how to protect myself from this gift of seeing. I saw much while I lived in New York. One day as I walked down 5th

Ave. I saw a male and female walking toward me, their steps in unison. I believe they were either demons or people filled with so much loathing and hatred that they were possessed. Their eyes were inhuman. They stared at me as they walked my way. No one else seemed to notice them. Another time on the subway, a possessed man came onto my car. He walked directly to me, sat down next to me, and stared at me with, creepy, colorless eyes. I was with my manager. This six foot six inch hulking man was terrified. Again, no one else noticed. The being followed me toward my home that night but my manager stuck by my side until it finally left. Another time in L.A. I was driving home on a very busy freeway. As I pulled into the slow flow of traffic, a person cut me off. The person harassed me incessantly driving in and out of the lane I was in. They drove up to my car at an unsafe pace then backed off. The occurrence was petrifying. So much so, I got off the freeway. The traffic on the off ramp was backed up. The car managed to follow me. While stuck on the ramp, the car started bumping me from behind. Eventually a woman, crazed, foam coming out of her mouth, stringy hair covering her face jumped out of the car and began beating my vehicle as she cursed my very existence. At one point she paused and looked me in the eyes. Again, her eyes were inhuman and her smile was full of malice.

The one through line in all these experiences was that I was in a very creative happy place in my life. I was at crucial turning points. In each situation, I faced the evil with confidence and faith. I looked them in the eyes, said my silent prayers, and thanked God for allowing me to understand I was on the right path. As they say, if evil shows its ugly face you're doing something right.

I believe that the world is a mysterious place full of good and evil. This belief keeps me on my toes. I don't spend too much time blaming or cursing GOD. I just continue to evolve and grow with awareness and thankfulness for the moments.

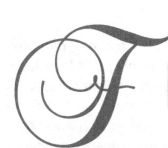

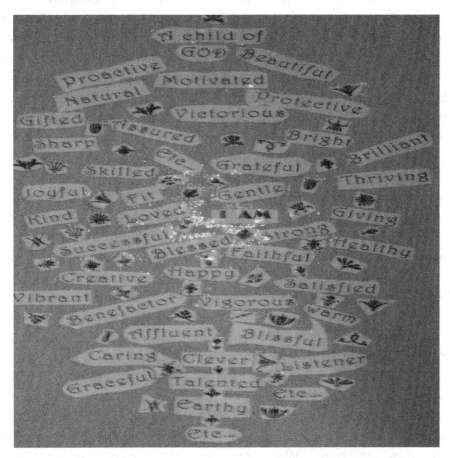

Status:
"Prayer"
December 10, 2014

One Way To Pray:

Dear Lord,

Please bless me; I beg of you. I don't like myself. Help me to be different. I hate my body. I can't stand to look in the mirror. But I love food. There's nothing wrong with that. I should be able to eat whatever I want! I hate exercise. It hurts and it takes too much time! So can you...just melt the pounds away? I know you can make that miracle happen. Speaking of miracles, will you please give me someone to love? I don't understand what is wrong with people. All I want is a good man. One that makes at least a three-figure salary, looks like the Rock, owns his house, and drives a couple of nice cars...And please make him drop all that football garbage and listen to me!? What I have to say is important. I need someone in my life that will listen! He'll also have to stop hanging out with that group of fools he calls friends. I won't like them...AND I won't want to spend every waking hour with his mamma! I need to be the woman in his life...AND please give me children that will obey me. I don't want any "Bebe" kids. Maybe you can send me a nanny when the time is right...BUT she can't be cute, Lord... maybe a "manny" would be better. And another thing... please destroy my enemies... all the people that don't agree with my way of thinking and my way of being need to go away somewhere else. Please make that happen. I beg you. Strike down all those people who are greedy and evil. They will never make it into Heaven. Lord, I need so much stuff. Will you please give me a lot of money so I can buy all the things I want? I want a new SUV, the newest and latest gadgets - I have to keep up with my girls... a mansion with a swimming pool somewhere warm... maybe two... I'll make sure I share with others... that is, people who are doing the right thing, living their lives in a righteous way. Lord... take care of my family, please. Save them from themselves. I don't understand why they just don't leave me alone. I know what I'm doing with my life. They don't know anything... Well... Anyway... That's all I need... for now. Thanks and Amen! Oh wait...Can you make these politicians do some work! I don't know what all the fuss is about. They're all corrupt anyway. Maybe you should strike them down, too! Amen!

Another Way To Pray:

Dear Lord,

What a wonderful GOD you are. I am so thankful for all your blessings. Thank you for waking me up this morning. I am grateful for my spiritual, mental, and physical health. Thank you so much for all the love I have in my life. Thank you for my family, friends, community, and the Earth. I appreciate how you take care of us all. I praise you for giving me all I need to glorify you. Thank you for all my gifts...I appreciate you bringing into my consciousness the gifts I have yet to recognize. Thank you for the journey I am on. Thank you for helping me to grow from every challenge. Thank you for helping me to be courageous when I face darkness. Thank you for helping me to understand, no matter how dark things seem, your light is penetrating. Thank you for spiritual, mental, and financial abundance. I appreciate the ability to humbly give back through gifts and works for your glory. Thank you for loving the world. I know you love us all...I know everyone is on his or her own course to you. Although I don't understand another man's path, thank you for helping me not to judge...But to love...Thank you for healing us all...Healing our world. Amen.

Although it may be difficult at times...I choose the latter prayer. Sometimes I want to complain to God...I want to be angry and whine...I want to be furious. "How can you let this world be such a horrible place? How can you let hunger and sickness ravage the land? How can you allow such nefarious corrupt people run our world?" I want to rage about how difficult it all is. I want to bitch about "what they did to me." But God is so good. I believe he listens to his disobedient, spoiled, rotten child with mercy... so I claim the goodness, compassion, and generosity of our supreme being. Although my challenging experiences seem endless, I recognize that I'm blooming and growing stronger and better through it all... I believe our world is growing better with every passing day. I see peace a comin'. I see change and a bursting forth of goodness and light. Is evil real? Probably... But GOD is more Tangible... Palpable... Authentic... Absolute...

Status:
"What's the problem? Just ask! You want that raise? I don't care what the economist says; just ask. You need a ride to work? Swallow your pride; just ask. You need to get out for date night with your partner? Go on and ask your family for help with the kids. You deserve a break; just ask. You need the higher power's intervention in a small seemingly inconsequential challenge? It wants you to flourish; just ask. Why are we so afraid to ask? Ego. What will they think of me? Will they think I'm weak? Will they judge me harshly? Is my need important enough? Yes... it is. If you don't ask, you will NEVER receive. All they can say is, no... "No is a two-letter word that gets to the point. I like that. Tell me no so I can move on and ask someone else. After you receive all the blessings you deserve, pay it forward. Just ask."
March 12, 2014

I'm Asking

I'm asking
I have no fear
I'm asking
My question's clear
I'm asking
I need you now
I'm asking
I want your vow
I'm asking
Will you be mine?
I'm asking
To make me shine
I'm asking
Can I be yours?
I'm asking
Forevermore

Status:
"FAITH"
January 21, 2014

I grew up in the church. Trinity United Methodist Church in Muncie, IN. What a phenomenal experience. The spiritual teachings were so important for my personal growth. Our church did tons of community outreach. We always celebrated Martin Luther King, Jr. Day... Even before it was a holiday (and those folks fought it – you know that!). I miss it sometimes... I haven't found the right fit in Illinois yet. I lived in Texas for a time and found a couple of great churches. I absolutely love One Community Church but started at Eternity Community Church. For some reason I'm reminiscing about my time in Texas. I remember one specific sermon. Maybe because this is apropos for how I'm feeling today. This is something I wrote at the time:

I went to church again today. I've been going to Haasan's church, Eternity Community Church. It's been a long time since I've been consistent going to a Christian gathering. The senior pastor, Kenneth Diggs, in a word, helps me. Every sermon I've heard feels as if it were conceived just for me. I always knew I wanted my daughter to be raised within the realm of some inspired faith. She is a very spiritual girl and has been since birth. She talks about God constantly and is very stirred by the Bible. I want to encourage that in her. I am very picky about what church I go to. I respect all faiths (although not all practices in the name of God) but I was raised Christian so that is what I want to pass on to Sophia. She can make her own decision for herself when she's old enough.

I had a difficult time finding the right church. Many of the most blessed churches have large congregations. That is great in a lot of ways. They help many people in this country and beyond. They definitely make a difference. But those mega churches make me feel like my family and I are inconsequential. I want to feel like we are a part of the family. I want to know the pastor and his wife. Then, some smaller churches tend to be far right conservative. These religious people have been the cruelest to me and mine. I have friends that I love who are Buddhists, gay, hip-hop performers, etc. I don't believe they are going to Hell because of their beliefs. I think everyone has their own path to God and no one should debase another because they don't believe the same way. That practice has chased me away from church far too often.

Now here I am...temporarily in Texas and I've found, through my brother, a church I'd like to be a part of. Dang! I'm leaving in June. It doesn't make sense to join. I hope I can find something comparable in Chicago. Who knows... maybe I'm finally ready to commit. Maybe that has been my problem all along.

Today Pastor Diggs struts his stuff in the cafeteria/auditorium at the Mooneyham Elementary School. They are temporarily here while their new establishment is being built a couple of blocks away. It's cool because it is only three minutes away from Haasan's home. Pastor Diggs is dressed in a sharp, black, three-piece suit. He is larger than life, although he stands only about 5'7" and carries a stocky carriage. He holds his congregation with penetrating bespectacled eyes and a stern mouth surrounded by a white goatee. His wife, Mother Diggs, is just as impressive as she stands off to his right, dressed in all white, her hair pulled back in a slick bun, supporting him with her joyous Amens and melodious moans of assent. He influences me again with his words of hope:

"You have to have a maturing faith... not just a superficial faith. Faith of a mustard seed is fine in the beginning... but it is a selfish faith, "God, thank you for blessing me. Please Lord, heal me... But when your faith matures, no matter what happens in your life you will believe and trust in God. Just like Shadrach, Meshach and Abednego, as they were on their way into the fiery furnace; they had faith. Just as Silas and Paul went to prison; they had faith. Just as Isaac was about to take his only son's life; he had faith. No matter how bad things look, you have to have faith. When enemies talk against you, you will praise the Lord. When life doesn't go your way, you will praise the Lord. When the doctor says there's nothing they can do, you will praise the Lord. When they take away your job, you will praise the Lord. When they smile in your face then throw you to the wolves, you will praise the Lord! Because you know that no matter the circumstances, God has a plan; he knows what he's doing. You will end up where you need to be. You will get there."

That's what I needed to think about that day. I need this reminder every day. I choose to dwell not on the fear but focus on faith.

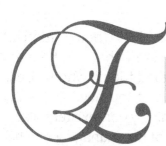

Ecstasy

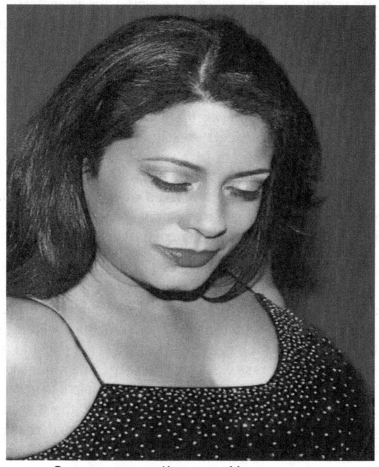

PHOTOGRAPH BY KATHLEEN MOSLEY

Status:
To Feel
May 5, 2014

107

We have many ways to survive challenges in our lives. Though some of these coping strategies work when we are children, they can be a deterrent to growth in adulthood. I have a very good friend, whom I'll call Teresa, who has gone through a very challenging journey. For many years she walked through life with a cold, seemingly non-existent heart. She had been sexually abused as a child. One of her managing mechanisms was to suffocate all feelings. She would not allow herself to get too close to anyone. Teresa believed that if she didn't expect anything from anyone, if she insulated her heart, she'd be sheltered from torment. She spent her entire early life cultivating this shield.

Teresa had it right. She could protect herself from hurting too intensely, but what she didn't count on was that she'd also stop having any sensations at all. Rarely did she feel the excitement of new love, the ecstasy of sexuality, the astonishment of a sunrise, or the comfort of close friendships. My friend went on like this for many years. Though Teresa had long-lasting relationships, they lacked energy and would invariably come to an end. She managed to maintain acquaintance with most of her exes because she never had enough passion to be angry.

After multiple broken associations, Teresa began to worry. She was growing older and less impenetrable. She started to feel the isolation she had created for herself. Teresa didn't have a single true friend. She had kept a thick defensive wall around her being for too long. She decided that to go on in this direction, would leave her sad and alone. A change was needed. Teresa was very intelligent. She rationally understood her choices. After reading numerous self-help books she determined to get some professional help. Fortunately, the therapist was amazing. She helped Teresa understand that her safeguarding behavior was stopping her from living life to the fullest.

As Teresa began to find her "feelings" she believed she had wasted much of her life. She became steadfast in her quest for "experience." With her liberated outlook, my friend finally found love. In years past, all of her choices for partnership had been safe ones. This lover reeked of danger. He had a wonderful spirit but he had made some unpopular decisions in his life. Everything about him seemed wrong for her. They came from different worlds. Teresa didn't care. Lover Man knew how to make her feel good with soothing, curative words and mind blowing eroticism. He mended Teresa's fractured heart. While breaching barriers with her exciting lover, Teresa finally came to terms with her childhood abusers. She was able to forgive. Her therapist had started her curing process but with Lover Man's brand of help, she began to heal.

Teresa was overwhelmed with her infatuation for Lover Man. She thrust herself into the relationship 100 percent. She was so full of ardor, she wrote him poetry, constantly encouraged him, gave him all the space he needed, was there when he was sick, held him when he worried about his future... she never asked a thing of him. In fact, this was Teresa's first love since the innocence of her first childhood relationship. She would have given him her everything. All she wanted in return was a little time. She was very independent and busy. She didn't have the lifestyle for an everyday union. She just wanted him to follow through when they made plans... for him to call when he said he would. He told her with ease how much he loved her, but he didn't have a clue how to show her. He didn't know how to give, how to share. He kept his life very secret. Lover Man usually only chose to see her for intimacy. In his way of thinking, this was love. The relationship was completely one-sided.

Teresa was confused by her own tolerance. She began calling it Karma. She thought her attraction to this selfish man was something she was spiritually working out. She wanted to feel, and she certainly did. She felt delight in his touch. She felt a thrill when he introduced her to new sensations. She felt bliss when he encouraged her. She felt... she also felt neglected. She felt crushing pain when he would stand her up. She felt intense anger when he behaved callously. He took advantage of her goodness. Eventually, he hurt her so deeply she screamed in pain. She felt... but she had to let him go.

Teresa found her heart. It was broken but not destroyed. She survived loving another but she finally understood she had to love herself... she will never forget Lover Man. In him, she exploded with emotion. With him, she came to life. She lived joy, pleasure, ecstasy, agony, hurt, and wretchedness. Teresa finally grieved him out of her heart but she knows she is at the beginning of a new path. Through Lover Man she found a profound love for herself. For that, she will always be thankful. Teresa was me.

Status:
"I am strong"
December 8, 2012

My Girl Down South

We were together at birth, she and I
Unaware of our tie we lived in ignorance
Of the gift of each other
We met, finally, at 4 years
What a joy she was to me
She made me feel connected
To the universe in a way
I didn't know existed
I saw stars when we mingled
My mind blew to pieces in delight
Bliss
Pure abandon
Loss of control, gladly
My girl down south and I were inseparable
Then came our 6th year
And with it an interruption to our harmony
Ignorance and hostility introduced
Curiosity and malice were their vices
My girl down south and I were terrorized
By furious
Instruments of infringement
Tools of trespass
Agents of anguish
A long held secret between us two
Fright became our new understanding

She couldn't endure the recollections
She went to sleep for 11 years
We met again in spring
She was feverish for association
And the light of awakening
Burned to attention
With a look from him
A most unlikely companion
My girl down south and I
Began to combust with expectation
We at long last began to interact once more
Our friendship rekindled
By way of his cornflower blue eyes
Until he sought advanced familiarity
More than we could give
We were alone, together again
We began to rediscover animation
No longer childhood play
We schemed to learn anew
My girl down south, and I
Then vicious discord offered itself
In devious barbarous brown hands
Venomous violation
Reprehensible ravishment
Brutal bullying
Holding each other during this onslaught
We vowed to never part
My girl down south, and I
We held fast
United in sorrow
Regret
Cold and near death
Until we inhaled the radiance
Of a healing soul
She restored our link to living
She mended our broken being

She melted our icy interior
We are now
Strong
Unbendable
Unbreakable
Alive
My girl down south, and I

Status:
"This is one of those days where the morning's events wore me out. I think I'll take a little nap."
January 15, 2014

I have been told that I am too nice. I've heard that all my life. I think that is hilarious because I can be the meanest person I know. I am very aware of my moods. When I am irritable I stay to myself. I don't want anyone to be mutilated by my sharp tongue. My daughter is the only person I can't avoid. We see each other daily so I'm hard to escape. I learned to give her fair warning. When I feel annoyance building I tell her, "Sophia, Mommy is ugly and irritable right now. Go find something to do." Very early on she learned to follow my instructions. When she was more naïve and rebellious she tested me. She was sorry. So was I.

The rest of the time, I am a pretty happy person. I like people and I love getting to know them. I don't do well in crowds but put me in an intimate setting and I'll get everyone in the room's life story. This gift has gotten me in some trouble. When a female is open and curious about a male, he very often thinks she is interested in him romantically. This scenario has played out so often in my life I have lost count. I wonder if women being nice to men they are not interested in is unusual. I hope not... but I wonder.

When I have been nice to men in power, they immediately assume I "want" them. I've had to be intensely careful. I desire a working relationship with great male directors and producers, but I have never been one to have sex with someone for work. That stance has made my chosen field a difficult road. The casting couch is real. Many men in power are used to women offering anything to get a job. I don't judge women who do this. Some women use their bodies as a commodity. They are welcome to. I just wish men wouldn't assume ALL women will do that. It sucks when I have to tiptoe around barely veiled sexual invitations. It wears me out to have to play dumb. I am a smart girl. I know when a man is insinuating what he wants from me, but I have to pretend ignorance so as to spare their feelings. Many men's egos get wrapped up in their sexual attractiveness. There have been times when I have not gotten a job because I wouldn't play the game. One time there was a very well-known director who told me directly that he would never hire me. He wasn't mean about it. He just said, "I'd rather have a mediocre actress that will be a freak, then have a great actress who ignores my tastes. Why do you think I do this stuff? It's not because I LOVE art... I love money and I love pussy. Film making gives me both." I was happy to know the truth.

I have had men "befriend" me hoping I will eventually give in and have sex with them. I've tried to fool myself into thinking that some of my "friends" were only that. Too often this has not been the case. These guy pals waited patiently in the wings hoping I'd one day be more. When they actually meet a woman they love, our friendship goes away. I have been hurt over and over. I've had very few true platonic relationships with men around my age.

Maybe as I get more wrinkles and let my hair finally go gray, I'll meet some buddies. One guy I know said, "Nope, C... as long as you can walk, there'll be men trying to get some. That's just men. They can't help themselves." I guess I'll just have to wait and see.

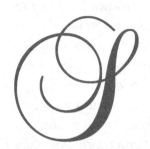

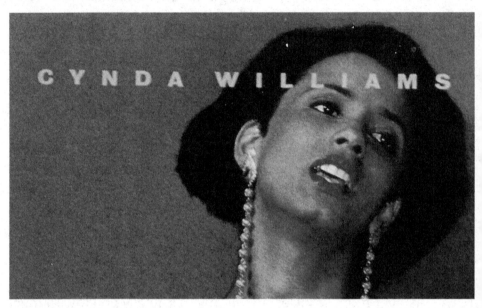

CYNDA WILLIAMS

Status:
"When life gives you a hundred reasons to cry, show life that you have a thousand reasons to smile." – Unknown
June 4, 2013

I developed a special skill when I was with a CERTAIN guy. In the beginning of our relationship I didn't have a thing to do. I wasn't auditioning; I'd only recently moved to L.A. and I had no friends. Certain was extremely jealous and didn't want me around his friends. He kept me at home in our little apartment unaccompanied where he could control my every move. I was so afraid of him I followed his orders. I really thought he would kill me if I didn't. He never hit me but he was always on the edge. He shook me up many times and would punch himself in his face if I disobeyed. He was 11 years older than me and I was so naïve. It never occurred to me that I could go outside and explore when he was off for hours at a time. I wasn't an adventurer so I had to learn to stay put, be quiet and alone. At first, I watched tons of TV. Court TV. I learned a lot. But I've never been a television girl. I needed books so I read and read and read. But that soon became a bore. I needed to have attention and the nature I loved; trees and plants, wind and ocean air. What was the point of living in sunny L.A. if I couldn't soak in the rays? So I started visualizing all those things on my uncomfortable futon, in my cramped bland bedroom. In my dreams I took long walks on the beach feeling the warm sand between my toes. I traipsed through the Red Wood Forest singing with the birds. I hiked up Runyun Canyon with my German Shephard and overlooked the smogless city. I made love to Certain in a lush king sized bed. I did all these magnificent things -- in my mind. What really happened went something like this:

I'm going to get me some tonight. I did my hair. It's kind of cute. My little Demi Moore cut sways into my eyes. Sexy. My make-up is all right. I'm no pro but I think it will do. After I bathed, I covered myself with rose scented lotion. I think he likes it. I'm wearing the pretty little yellow do-dad I found at Victoria's Secret. It is lacy and barely covers my unmentionables. I know I look good. I even got some yellow pumps to go with it when I was back in Muncie. Before this prison... Oh well... here goes.

He is sitting on the bed reading a script he wrote -- again. I don't know why he's stressing it. It's brilliant. I should know. I helped him write it. But he's a perfectionist and I don't question him. He's an amazing writer. I'm just a beginner. He has on cute white boxers and a wife beater (kind of appropriate – stop thinking that way). He's got on his glasses. I love his glasses. He looks so studious and that's my thang. I walk over and stand in front of him. He doesn't notice. "Certain, what you doin'?" He says, "What you think?" I sit next to him. I snuggle his throat. He nudges me aside. "Certain, I want to make love." He says, "I ain't in the mood. Maybe later." Well damn...

There never was a later. Crazy, jealous, MF. It was my fault, though. I should never have been with that fool in the first place, but you know...

115

we'd had sexual intercourse and that stuff was good, so I had to move in with him! I'm monogamous but stupid. Call it religious conditioning. Little did I know he was out sleeping with everything that walked. But he wouldn't touch me. No way. The last night we lived apart was the last time he made love to me. It was terrible for my self-esteem. I thought there was something appallingly amiss with me. There had to be. Maybe, I wasn't good enough. He paid more attention to the gay boys that flirted with him outside our West Hollywood apartment:

Certain and I are going to dinner and a movie. We're seeing Dances With Wolves. I'm very excited because I've heard so much about it. I can't believe Kevin Costner has directed such an important story. I look forward to seeing it. Certain and I take the elevator to the parking garage. He looks adorable tonight. He's got on torn jeans, a black tee and a leather jacket. His hair is long and in a ponytail under his baseball hat. I wish he'd just cut it off. So what he's balding? He's a beautiful man. He doesn't need hair. His 195-pound frame is so manly. I'm not usually so attracted to white men, but he's different. He is such a man's man. Just like my daddy. So what he's a bit prejudiced? I can't believe he's with me, sometimes. He doesn't always seem to like black people; certainly not our culture. If we fight, that's what it's about, "that stupid Jazz music" or "those pieces of garbage movies those people make."

Anyway we walk to his classic convertible Mustang. He gets there first and revs the engine telling me to "hurry up." I do. A pretty little body builder type walks up to Certain and says, "Oooo, he roars." Certain chuckles with his charismatic behind and the guy almost faints. It's like these fools don't see me standing there. They are so rude.

We ate a silent dinner. I wonder what's going on with him. There is no pleasing him. The waiter, who was an attractive Latino, was very nice to us. To US. Certain insisted I was crafting a liaison with the man! Just because I said please and thank you, I was flirting. What a freak.

We are at the movie. It is wonderful. I just love looking at all these gorgeous Native Americans, the men and women alike. The cinematography is outstanding and the script is so well crafted I cry at its beauty. Certain asks me what I'm crying about. Why the hell did I tell him?! He just leaves the theater stomping, huffing and puffing all the way. Well, I'm glad he's gone. Maybe he'll think a little bit about how stupid he's being while I watch this masterpiece in tranquility. I sit there and enjoy every bit of it.

Certain's gone! He not only left the screening room but he left me here with no transportation, in Glendale, all alone. I guess I'll call his friends. They'll pick me up, I think. They are his friends. What have I gotten myself into?!

Status:
"What a day...All I can do is pray."
April 17, 2013

Whose Son are you?

Come in my house with no regard?
Yanking strings, acting hard?
You think I'm weak?
Oh no I'm strong.
I won't lie down.
You've got it wrong.
Whose son are you?

Whose son am I?
Can't see her face.
She went away and left this place.
Never knew my mama's care.
She left for good without a prayer.

You were a fool to show up here.
And I still say, might disappear.
I won't forgive and can't forget
Your arrogance and silly threats.
Whose son are you?

Whose son am I?
I miss his smile.

117

My daddy left a lonely child.
Went up above and far away.
And I became the world's cliché.

Whose son are you?
Creating scenes.
Whose son are you?
Crude and obscene.
Whose son are you?
Hurt and demean.
Whose son are you?
Don't you see queens?

Talk down to us then use your fist.
Scream, shout, and cuss,
Now I'm pissed.
Recognize we're bold and brave
Can't come in here and misbehave.
Whose son are you?

Whose son am I?
I'm no one's son.
The world has taught me,
To trust no one.
Not one kindness
Was shown to me.
I just survived
So let me be.

Status:
That Special Bond With Their Private Parts
March 30, 2014

Let me start by saying that I adore men. I know I've said that before but
I have to be clear. Men are very curious creatures. I love to study them.
I delight in trying to get into their heads and examine how they perceive
the world. I bask in writing male characters. When others read my work

and say they "believed" my masculine personas, I am very pleased. I know I'll never truly live in the universal man mind, but taking the time to understand them has made me very forgiving.

In all cases but one: All my life I have been dealing with men that find pleasure in trying to shock me with their "member." As a child, living in Chicago, when I would walk to school there were numerous times when some guy would approach me and begin massaging his naked personal property. These men usually have a sly, leering countenance. They look forward to seeing a young child's fright. It happened so often that I got desensitized to the experience. The last time it occurred, I was walking home from Northside, my high school in Muncie, IN. My building was next to an elementary school. An old, shriveled up grandfather sat in his pick-up with the door open. He was waiting with baited breath, yanking and stroking, as the little ones made their way home. This was a final straw for me. I started yelling at the goof ball. "You nasty sicko, leave these kids alone!!! Get outta here!" Regrettably, he was turned on by my response to him. He proceeded to follow my path as I made my way home. I had to switch up my direction to lose him. I was terrified. Of course I told my father (he still lived in Chicago) who promptly drove to Muncie to help me deal with this situation. Unfortunately, I didn't have the presence of mind to memorize the pervert's license plate. I was just trying to save myself from possible molestation. I reported him to the police and the school officials. He had been sexually harassing children for about two years. I don't think they ever caught the jerk.

I understand men have a special bond with their private parts. It is their unique physical trait. Stimulation brings them unimaginable pleasure. They have their own special personalities. I get it. It is a powerful tool in the procreation needed in our world. There is nothing wrong in my opinion for a man to appreciate his distinct gift, but when he uses his organ to terrorize, molest, and violate someone, he has a sickness that needs to be healed.

My daughter and her friends had their first introduction to a corrupted fellow who had to reveal his stuff to them. It was online. He continuously sent them pictures of it. Sophia blocked him but he managed to bypass her attempts at banishment and showed her his pride and joy. I was not in town when this happened. She was embarrassed and afraid. I, of course, wanted to find the bastard and break it off but that was impossible. At least she didn't have to see it live and in person.

I proceeded to try to take the sting out of the experience. I told my daughter this: "The penis is nothing but a body part. Just like there are many people with different shapes and sizes – fat, thin, short, tall, white, black, etc., penises come in many different forms. They are a natural and beautiful part of the hu-'man' body. They have numerous labels: dick, prick, hot dog, sausage, big boy, little boy, rod, cock, putz, dong, horn, joint, knob and many more. Those are words sometimes meant to offend but they are just letters put together. Don't be embarrassed by these monikers. You win the battle if you can manage not to be upset by symbols of ignorance. Phalluses are not to be feared... they're just anatomy. If deviants are attached to them, they are the problem. So if a jerk sends you a photo of his stuff, recognize the beauty of God's creation, delete it, and let it go. If a degenerate approaches you in person, run, scream, then tell your daddy, uncles, cousins, and grandfather. If the fool is lucky enough to hide from them, he better pray Mommy don't find him."

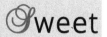

*S*weet

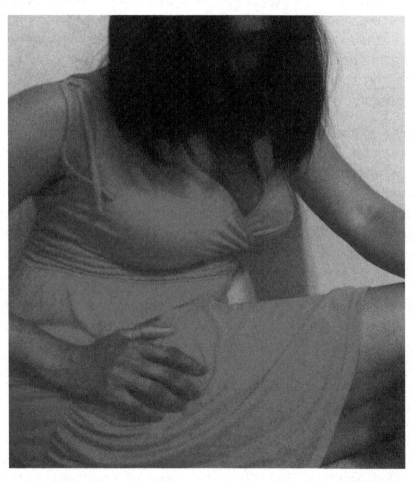

Status:
"Sweet Cyn"
March 18, 2014

I'm not always "Sweet Cyn."

I work very diligently at being positive. It is a constant trial. My inbred way to deal with challenges is with anger and depression. I witnessed these behavioral patterns as a child.

I love my parents very much. They have been amazing to my siblings and I. I believe the success we've been able to acquire in our lives started with them. They taught us strength in times of adversity, loyalty, and perseverance. They have been role models for us in many positive ways. I wouldn't want anyone else in his or her places. They were great parents but not necessarily a great couple. They had a very rocky marriage right from the start. Dealing with physical illness and outside forces made their delicate union overwhelming at times.

Daddy's job was scary and dangerous. Being CPD, he was out patrolling the streets of Chicago when gang violence was starting to percolate. Racism ran rampant in the department and progressing to more lucrative and empowered positions was very difficult. Add insult to injury, my dad was ill with hyperthyroidism. That condition makes you feel as if your body is always quaking, your nerves are constantly on edge, and your heart is beating out of control. It is a wonder he didn't lose his cool on his job. That shows his strength.

My mother dealt with discrimination daily. She was a white woman who dared to marry a black man in the 60s. A time of BLACK POWER; Black women loathed her. White people despised her. My mother also was handicapped from years of battling polio. She was often in the hospital with yet another surgery. Pain will make you mean. My mom has withstood pain her entire life. That shows her resilience.

It's no wonder they argued often. Or should I say, Daddy yelled and Mommy stewed which made him yell, which made her stew more. Anger and depression: That is how they dealt with problems at times. I was a willing student. All children learn the most from what they see at home. I know my parents weren't thinking, "I want Cindy to throw her fist into the wall. Let me show her how it's done. I want Cindy to roll up in a ball and sob for hours then lay as if comatose for more." No. They were young. They didn't understand that they were teaching me how to cope in an unhealthy way. I think parents forget their power. "Do as I say, not as I do" does not work. Children always do what you do. Always. I did. My parents got better. They learned to communicate. It took me a while to follow their lead. Now I'm trying to help Sophia to stop coping in the horrible ways I have modeled!

When I voice my pain, I stop feeling it. It doesn't get pushed deep inside where it then explodes out onto the people I love the most. I don't like myself when I'm enraged. I abhor myself when I want to lie in the bed with self-pity. So I get it out. I prefer Sweet Cyn. My world is better for it.

Status:
"Who knew pink would grow on me."
April 25, 2014

Pink Panties

I so adore my pink panties
Who knew that pink would grow on me?
The color of femininity
Afraid of the attention, see?
I've long denied that side of me
Now I'm primed, ready, and free
To embrace the girl in me
I accept my beauty in my
Cupid cotton v-kinis complimenting my shade of brown
I admit I'm precious in my
Raspberry Sherbet jersey bikinis cooling my hot skin
I believe my exquisite magnificence in my
Iris Mauve, satin, hipsters tickling away my blues
I declare my radiance in my
Wineberry lace thongs whispering secrets revealed
I so adore my pink panties
Who knew that pink would grow on me?
The color of femininity
Afraid of the attention, see?

I've long denied that side of me
Now I'm primed, ready, and free
To embrace the girl in me

Status:
"Today I'm feeling girlie. I wish the weather would let me wear a sun-
dress. Hey, Snow! GO AWAY until another day! Like December."
April 15, 2014

I am a tomboy: Plain and simple. I grew up primarily with knuckle-
headed boys. I ran, fought, and scraped my knees with the best of
them. In the beginning I never cared about my apparel. As long as I
could keep up with my brothers, that's all that mattered. That changed
when I became a student. In school, your class is determined by the
brands you wear, the quality of your clothing, and the stores you
bought them in.

We could not afford expensive wear. Food and a home were more important to my parents so I held tightly to my boyishness. It was cheaper.
Beautiful things cost more. Besides, I always thought I was ugly, anyway. I didn't even try to fit into the pretty world.

Out of envy, I developed an unwarranted disdain for "girlie-girls." I
couldn't stand their prissiness, despised floral patterns, and scoffed at
ruffles and wearing dresses (unless I was forced for church). For a long
time I made myself believe that those types of females were the enemy.
I imagined they looked down their noses at anyone that wasn't like
them; that wasn't pretty like them.

I wore hand-me-downs, was never in the current style, so I had no at-
tachments to fashion. I wore basic jeans and solid colored shirts or
sweaters depending on the season. My underwear was cotton and
practical. My bras were basic. My shoes were no nonsense.

As I grew older I did manage to create my own funky style. I never wore brand names, but my Aunt Spring taught me how to liven up my unadorned jeans. I would create elaborate designs with needlepoint on them. I also added pizzazz with cheap accessories, colorful socks, and bright leg warmers. Those were affordable. I sometimes wore interesting hats. I needed them to cover up my bad hair.

Neither my white mother nor my black aunts or grandmother had a clue how to do my hair. Mixed race locks were a challenge to all of them. My tresses took a long time to grow because my mother would put grease on my scalp like all the black moms. Unfortunately, my hair follicles retaliated for that abuse by not growing. When I finally started learning how to style my own hair, it grew but remained unhealthy. Why? For the longest time I got press and curls. I still have the burnt hair smell in my nostrils. Later, I would ask the local beauticians to treat my mane with harsh chemicals. I wanted the "jheri curl" look like the other girls. I had no idea that I had under all those chemicals, grease, and baby oil, naturally curled ringlets. I ended up burning my head bald.

It wasn't until I moved away to NYC that I started to get in touch with my girlie side. When I started to make money I discovered that I did like womanly things. I started to care even more about how adornments made me feel on the inside. After I met a phenomenal hairdresser who taught me how to do my own hair, I wore it natural. Once the funds were coming in I started to buy attractive clothing. I found that I loved pretty matching lingerie. I became a shoe and purse fanatic. I still had doubts that I'd be anything but unpleasant but I could cover it up with beautiful fabrics and sharp designs. I never became a spendthrift though. I remained frugal by shopping in thrift shops. I was able to find lovely and unique garments.

Nowadays, I have distinct moods when it comes to what I wear. Some days I'm in black from head to foot. Other days I beam in floral sundresses. Most often I live in leggings and tanks unless I have an audition. When you have a child, all your resources are funneled to their needs. But I will sock away some money for lovely lingerie. I prefer pink panties and bras. Even though no one else can see them, I know they're there. When I take off the costume of my daily grind, I am met with femininity; and then I feel pretty and realize I am.

PINK PANTIE CONFESSIONS

*I*dealism

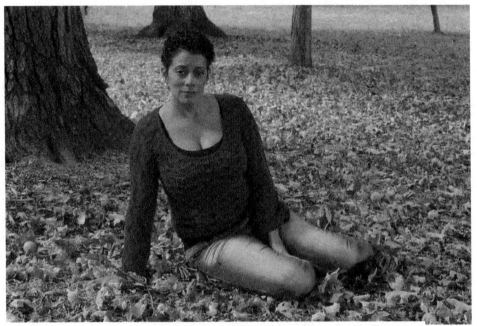

PHOTOGRAPH BY PAUL TROXELL

Status:
"Thinking positive thoughts for those in fear, praying thankful prayers for those in need, meditating on supernatural prosperity for those who can't see their way to the light beyond Earthly sight. I'm shifting my communication with the Divine to one of gratitude for you and yours and me and mine. Will you do the same today? Thank you, God. Thank you, you."
October 1, 2013

I've spent too much time wishing for things. I've wished for love, for money, for my dream house, and many other seemingly simple desires.

The problem is the "wishing" part. Wishing infers lack. The Universe doesn't understand my meaning if I'm not clear. If I say, "I wish for...," I indicate to the Universe that I don't have something. All the attention is on the lack. It says, "Okay, let me keep giving this girl what she asks for. She's focusing on the fact that she has never owned a house. Let's keep it that way! She says she has no love. Let's leave her lonely for a while longer. She barely makes ends meet. She must like living that way. The minute we start to claim with faith what we desire is when God agrees with us. Sometimes she blesses us with more than we think we deserve.

"I thank you God for the new, creative friendship I have in my life." I get three new friends or more. "I thank you God for love in my life." A dog shows up on my doorstep. "Thank you God for my new lover." I get one. What kind will he/she be? If I'm not specific, I may end up getting a jackass that is a one-night stand. "I want a great male friend that motivates me; I want a gentle male friend that is a great lover; I want a successful male friend that has a good job that I can travel with." I could end up with three male friends that do each thing I desired instead of one with all. I have to claim what I desire with clarity and preciseness. Then quiet my mind and mouth and let God do what he does.

Status:
"Amazing how life can give you a life-shattering challenge then turn around and mend you up so much better than before. Keep your heart on what you have, not what you lose... then life will give you more blessings than you could ever imagine."
October 15, 2014

When I Met You

When I met you
My heart I held so closed and safe
Opened wide
Like a deep and untouched cavern
Revealed to God's Sun for the first time
Although you didn't seem to see me
I dove deep within your being and
I felt the purity of your soul

128

You didn't know I was there, did you?
When I met you
My dark skies yawned
Unobstructed for the first time
Yes: The gloomy clouds disintegrated
Into particles of hope
My waning moon
Suddenly became FULL of the
Possibilities
Although you didn't seem to feel me
I felt my heart intermingled with yours
And knew all was finally as it should be
You didn't know you became my air, did you?
When I met you
I knew you were ALL
All I've ever wanted
When I met you

Status:
Well, I Wanna be Like Joshua
May 22, 2014

Have you ever been in bondage? Any kind? Have you been imprisoned, guilty or innocent? Have you ever been enslaved by choices in your life?

How about being a serf to addictions? Maybe drugs, cigarettes, fatty foods, sugar, alcohol, rage driving, unhealthy relationships, depression, obsessions, possessions, damaging lack of self-esteem, hate, anger, racism, prejudice, status, a noxious job, wacko friends, extreme sports? I think most everyone has been attracted to something self-destructive. I don't know if we make these choices because it is a self-imposed life lesson or that we're contented with sickness, pain, and suffering.

Recently, I watched one of my favorite animated movies...again...for the umpteenth time. DreamWorks' "The Prince of Egypt" moves, motivates, and enlightens me with each viewing. I experienced it in a different way this time. I was cleaning alone, as I often do, but I wanted company so I turned the movie up and listened as I worked. I heard lyrics, dialog, tone and nuance I'd missed before. Since most people of the Jewish, Christian and Muslim faith know the story of Moses and the Exodus (if you don't, you should read it. It's one of the greatest stories ever told) I won't repeat it here. This great history of a people got me to thinking about the different types of self-imposed oppression I've tolerated in my life.

I've fought many battles with addictions (none of the heavy hitters, so don't start). I'll speak of one. Many years ago I was in an unhealthy relationship (I've had a few – addiction, see?). I knew the minute I started this excursion that it was going to be difficult. The guy (Certain - remember him?) thought he loved me but he did not. He barely liked me and I knew it. We were worlds apart in every way. We shared intimacy and property. We lived together...all the things grown-ups do...but I was no grown up. I was raised to "stay by your man" through thick and thin. I felt trapped. I was so stuck that it took him cheating, lying and finally leaving me before I could let him go. Like Jewish people, I had grown comfortable with my misery. Remember how they argued about the pros and cons of slavery?

At least they had their hovels, food and the closeness of family. No matter they were mistreated, loathed, violated, and ENSLAVED! Now here comes Moses trying to stir stuff up!

Affliction has a level of security. We understand it. There are no surprises.

So what happens when WE finally march OUT of our Egypt? Will we be strong and courageous like Joshua? Or will we complain, be faithless and wander in the wilderness for 40 years? Will we watch God provide and yet cry out, "I want to go back to torment?" I think that's why when we get out of our cages, the road is so precarious. We seek the familiar no matter how horrible; no matter that God is pointing us to freedom and the Promised Land. Fear and laziness stops us from going into Canaan to fight the battle to get the happiness we deserve. Well I wanna be like Joshua. If the other Israelites had his strength, courage and faith they would have strolled directly from Egypt into their new home of plenty. That's how I want to do it every time I break out. Just like Joshua.

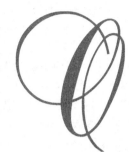

PINK PANTIE
CONFESSIONS

Outpour

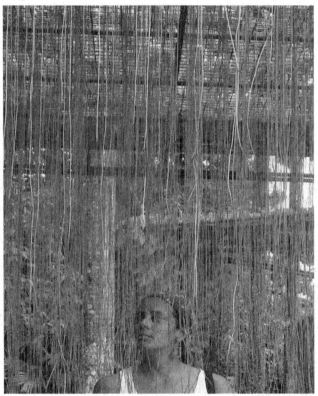

Status:
"Sometimes agitating incidents occur that stall your momentum. Don't let the frustration triumph. Stop, breathe, rest in the pause, and let your awareness soar. You might find that the direction you were madly dashing toward would have taken you to an exciting... dead end."
February 28, 2014

131

It drives me crazy when I am seemingly on the road to success and something happens to bring it all to a halt. It might be a positive something, or not; but I get very pissed off about it. If I feel something is working, I can be very stubborn about changing.

I have learned to chill in those situations. Not every road is mine. Not every role, job possibility, or relationship is the best situation for me. My vision of my future might be too small. I know I can't see the big picture. I can't fathom all the possibilities. There are times when I have to let go of "doing it my way" and let my universe expand.

If I had had my own way, I would still be doing small movies and sporadic television roles. Life didn't allow it. The economy crashed, work dried up. I was nearing my 40's (death for actresses in Hollywood) and I had my baby girl. I could no longer do the same thing the same way. I've been writing my entire life but only for me, myself, and I – my words, my property. I was extremely selfish about sharing. I kept hearing in my soul "write for others." What else was I going to do? I may fight those voices but they eventually win in the end. I started writing for the public. I've only recently begun to think about publishing, but if you're reading this I guess I've moved to the next phase.

I love acting and pray I do a lot more of it...I also have a voice beyond the characters I play. My career so far has been beneficial in giving me a platform for something more important. God ain't going to let me "do the easy." I've been forced to move and shift in another direction. So here I sit, at my computer, writing these words. I love every minute of it.

Status:
"Someone I knew and loved slipped into my consciousness today. I finally allowed myself to grieve. I know he's in a better place. I love you D."
October 16, 2013

Fill Me Up

Oh what a night.
The residue of you still holds me tight.

The memory of your touch
Makes me feel so much...

I am willing to sacrifice
All the love I have inside.
Is it all in my mind?
Or do you find
What I think I've found
When I'm loving you.
> Cause you fill me up.
> You fill me up
> And how my cup
> Runs over
> With the love I feel for you
> You fill me up.
> I'm giving up.
> My heart belongs to you.

Your voice makes me quiver.
When I think of you I shiver.
I still feel your fingertips
I dream of your kiss on my lips.
> Cause you fill me up.
> You fill me up
> And how my cup runs over
> With the love I feel for you.
> You fill me up.
> I'm giving up.
> My heart belongs to you.

I never thought I'd know love
Till I met you
And my heart grew
Deep inside of me.
Now I know that there is no one
Who will find me
And will thrill me
So tenderly.

Cause you fill me up.
You fill me up
And how my cup runs over
With the love I feel for you.
You fill me up.
I'm giving up.
My heart belongs to you.

Lyrics and melody – Cynda Williams; Music – Dee Harvey

Status:
This Time of Year
December 20, 2013

The Christmas Season is my most cherished time of the year. There are so many things I love about it. For one thing, I adore the multi-colored strings of lights that festoon the homes. Winter is such a dark time. The lighting festively brightens the nights. Christmas trees hold a special place in my heart. I prefer living trees but I always feel bad about killing one for a month's enjoyment. It just doesn't feel right. For this reason we have a fake tree. I have tenderness for ornaments old and new. I collect at least one unique pretty thing a year. I like tinsel, as messy as it is. The lights on the tree glisten against the silver and/or gold. I absolutely enjoy the seasonal smells – pine, cinnamon and cookies. Eggnog with spice and a shot of whiskey turns my tongue into a flavor explosion. I watch every Christmas animated film I can, preferably in real time. No DVR action. I want to watch them as they are aired, just like I did when I was a child. "A Charlie Brown Christmas" is my favorite. I watch "It's a Wonderful Life" and "Miracle on 34th Street" yearly. I delight in Christmas music. Not so much the pop tunes but the classical choral and instrumental orchestrations.

My favorite part of Christmas is spending time with family. It is a wonderful time when we can be with my parents, our brothers, sisters, nieces, nephews, cousins, play cousins, etc. We don't get to do it often considering the miles between us. Sometimes I feel for Sophia being an only child in our home (she does have a lovely half-brother, but he's grown and isn't close by). Christmas is about connections. When we were growing up, my extended family would usually come to Chicago to celebrate with us. My grandparents, aunts, uncles, and cousins would all cram into our house. It was such a thrilling time. Whatever challenges or disputes we had were put aside. If there was an issue, you tabled it until December 26th. The family would invariably spread out in groups after the greetings were made. The women would prepare the feast the entire day of Christmas Eve. They could cook!!! Especially my grandma. Every dish she made came out tasting like perfection. My Aunt Annalee was a fabulous pastry chef. The pies were delicious. The men would usually crash in front of the TV loudly cheering for whatever basketball or football team was playing. My dad kept the wood fireplace hot. The kids played either in our finished basement or up in the bedrooms. Our parents would often throw us outside with the dogs for hours to tire us out. I'm sure they needed some reprieve from the constant yelling, laughing, and fighting. For years I was the only girl so I got to intermingle amongst any of these groups.

Gifts were exciting but they weren't the central theme of the holiday in those days. Every Christmas morning the tree would be almost buried with gifts because there were so many of us but we only got two gifts at most.

I grew up in the Christian church so the account of Jesus' birth was one I was very familiar with. My grandfather was a pastor and made sure we knew "the reason for the season"- It's about the gift of Jesus' life. I revered the nativity story. I'd often imagined how difficult the times must have been for Mary and Joseph. My poppa never sugarcoated the truth. He would explain the religious dogma of the times – the rules Jewish people were meant to follow. It was a miracle that Mary wasn't stoned or at least flogged for saying she was the mother of the Messiah and pregnant by God. She had to be VERY brave and Joseph had to be the kindest man on Earth.

This was the usual Christmas Eve night ritual: The children would look under the tree forlornly. There were a few gifts sprinkled about but nothing substantial. We were always exhausted by 8 p.m. We would usually eat something light and easy. The heavy eating was always saved for Christmas day. We'd sit in front of the TV watching a Christmas special but we couldn't really get into it. The anticipation was just too overwhelming. Then the dreaded bedtime would be announced, "Go to bed! Now! Do not pass go, go directly to bed!" Someone always cautioned us that if we got up, Santa WOULD NOT come and Daddy couldn't help but warn us, "If anybody gets up, you ALL will get a whippin'!" So off to bed we'd go, every year, except when I turned 8. I suffered from insomnia then, just like now. I decided to brave Santa's wrath and my daddy's belt and see what in the world happened after 9 o'clock p.m. on Christmas Eve. I made sure neither of my snot-nosed brothers or crazy cousins followed me as I tiptoed down the stairs. What I saw was a shock. Some of the adults danced around the living room to the soulful hits from the time – something from Earth, Wind, and Fire, I think. Everybody toasted and drank something. It wasn't eggnog, that's for sure. Daddy had a brown bag of barbecued rib tips and white bread. He had sauce dripping down his mouth as he laughed at something my Uncle King said. Aunt Sodiqa was doing some African dance moves, as usual.

Poppa shook his head and smiled. I crept down the stairs and into the kitchen. No one was there. I peeked into the dining room. Mommy and all the other adults surrounded the dining-room table busily wrapping gifts. So that was how so many gifts ended up under the tree! Wait...No Santa?! I stood there quaking with anger for a minute. They lied to me!!!! But my angst only lasted a moment. I had always recognized my poppa dressed up like Santa on Christmas mornings past. My daddy and uncles were his elves. I just assumed they were Santa's representatives. What I saw here was so much better than a fat, old, stranger sliding down my chimney.

The Williams house was filled with love and affection. Our parents LOVED us so much they performed this tradition every year. It couldn't have been easy hiding all these toys, sneaking around playing it cool. Keeping secrets. I couldn't wait until I grew up so I could play my part in this side of the Christmas drama. After taking all this joy in, I finally took myself to bed and slept soundly. I'm not sure I've ever felt that enveloped in safety and goodness again.

So, yes, I'm one of those Christmas lovers. My prayer is that each one of you feels peace, safety, and love Christmas 2013 and beyond.

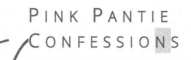

Nepotism

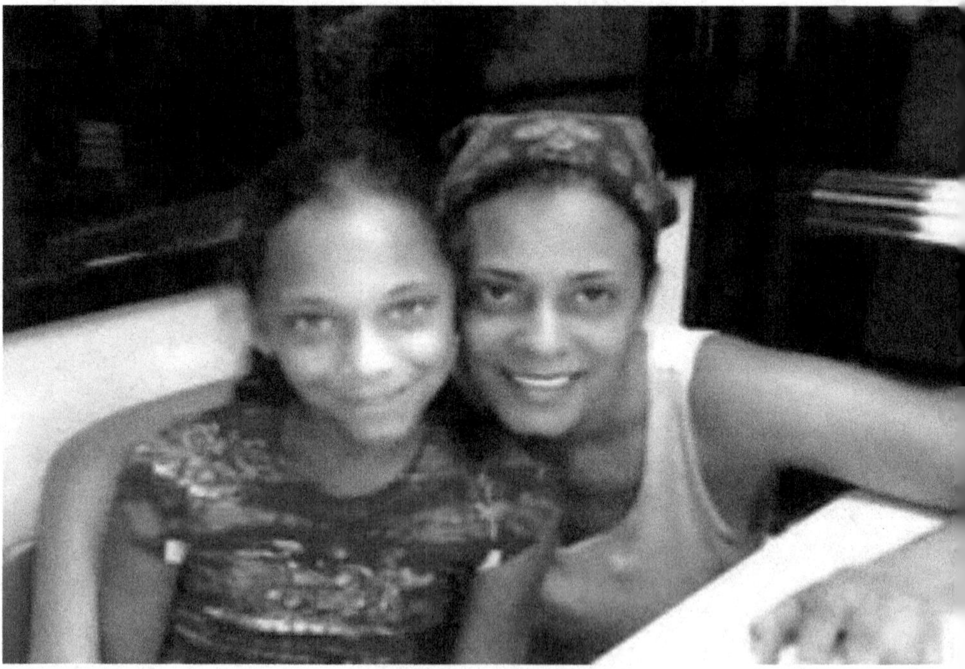

Home Schooling Sophia

Status:
Home Schooling
December 12, 2013

This morning as I got up at 5:45 a.m. to take my daughter to school I was a bit cantankerous. I was tired. I got to bed late because I couldn't sleep. My bedroom feels like a sauna. I have always preferred a cool space for sleep. The problem is, the rest of the place will be chilly if I keep the temperature too low so I have to turn on the ceiling fan, the floor fan, and open the window in order to sleep. This morning as I awakened I was lying in a pool of perspiration. Gross!!! I heard my daughter stir and I wished I could sit in a cool bath and gradually wake up. The crazy thing is, it is one degree outside!

My daughter came into my room. "Time to get up Mom. I've got to be to school an hour early for the pancake breakfast." EEEEKKKK! So I rolled out of my sweaty sheets and started my day. As I washed off the night's grime I started remembering when we lived in Singapore with my husband. I always woke up this way. The difference was, I didn't have to take Sophia to school...I was home schooling her. When that memory crossed my mind I stopped feeling sorry for myself:

Sophia began home schooling this week. OKAYYYY...

Sophia is attending the prestigious K12 International Online School. Phenomenal! Excellent! Awesome! The coolest!

It is a rigorous and exciting program. I am sure Sophia will return to traditional school fully enriched and ahead of the game. The program uses interactive online games and lessons; offline texts and workbooks, and a collection of provided materials. Our office looks like a small classroom. Her core courses are: Science, History, English (language skills – grammar usage and mechanics – literature skills, read aloud/independent reading, writing, and spelling) and Math. Her extra courses are Art and Chinese Mandarin. Wow! The school is a blessing for her!

It was not our intention to put Sophia into this kind of program but the circumstances of our arrival (the late date and the ridiculous financial expectation for starting fees) gave us very little choice.

The entire process for enrollment of a foreigner into the Singapore public school system is extremely complicated. There are many assessments to take; the concentration on tests are monumental – even more so than at home (and that's saying something). Spots in higher education are sparse so the competition is great.

The first of these tests for advancement starts at 3rd grade. A child's life can be forever affected if they do not do well at this stage. A small percentage of students that qualify are placed in the best institutions the government can offer, while the majority of the children whose scores are below a certain point are parceled off to less effective schools. They rarely catch up. And it goes on. So, THAT option was out.

Then there's the International School option. We loved the schools we toured. They teach from a Baccalaureate Standard. It is a hands-on, flexible approach where independent learning is promoted. The classes are fun. The students come from all over the world. Tests are important but not the be-all-to-end-all. BUT to get in -- huh! Expensive, expensive, expensive!!! They want MOST of the cash up front. They want your child's life's history (transcripts, proof of identity documents, letters of referral, etc.) with a promise in blood to abide by their rules of engagement. The requirements rival the Ivy Leagues. So THAT was out!

Sigh, sigh. K12 International Online HOME SCHOOL! BUT what the K12 CONTRACTORS didn't tell us, before they took our money, is that the "learning coach" (me!) is really the individual teaching this stuff. They claimed that I would only have to participate 20% of the time. But my friends, that is bogus! Yes, there is an on-line teacher BUT she is simply a resource for answering questions that I am too daft to understand.

The teacher will communicate with Sophia once every two weeks at most. There are online virtual classes, class connect sessions, where Sophia can join other students and the teacher to go through certain subjects. But her teacher lives in Dubai, which is five hours earlier than Singapore. She'd have to get that kind of help AFTER working 7-8 hours already, so that leaves me. I am participating ALL DAY! ALL 7-8 hours (recess, two short breaks, craft services and fine dining included). Sophia can work independently - I insist on it. But she needs guidance much of the time. So, let's say I wanted to get "Physical" with one of my Buns of Steel DVDs, FORGET IT! No time. So I have to get my buns up at 5:15 a.m. to get my sweat on. So here we go. Who knew I'd become this kind of teacher so far into my life. An acting coach, I saw that. Maybe even a professor of acting at some prestigious university, but a 4th grade teacher? Heck no!

I gotta tell you, though, our most daunting challenge is this brand new dynamic to our relationship. Sophia and I get along very well for the most part. She communicates openly with me and I guide her the best I can. I am also the disciplinarian. My husband has the job of soothing Sophia's injured ego when I push her too roughly. I try not to be too hard-core but I do have some of my daddy and a lot of my grandma in me. Transitioning to the teacher/student mode is very different. A different kind of respect is required. We are BOTH working on this subtle transition. It will take time. Ultimately, it will make us closer. In the meantime, she'll try not to break down crying when she's frustrated and I'll try not to raise my voice.

We are being creative. We are making things happen.

What am I to learn at this juncture of my life? What is the lesson here, oh Lord: How to spell "establishment?" How to find mountain ranges on a map? How to divide fractions? I guess I'll have to be patient and see. Gotta love the adventure!

Status:
"You may not have the love you want, but you have the love you need, because it is the love you have. It's all love."
February 19, 2014

God's Grace

The doctor smiled, gave me my child
Then I met God's grace

I never knew that I was blue
Until I saw your face

I couldn't feel, nor did I heal
And I would not admit it

I didn't know I had a hole
Until you came and filled it

141

The sun burned bright, the moon at night
All came to life with you

You were my world, my lovely girl
You were my true breakthrough

So I will aim to do the same
Be mother and your friend

So for a start, I'll give my heart
I'll love you till the end

Status:
The Singapore Botanical Gardens
January 6, 2014

There are record shattering temps today. With wind chill it is 45 below. Businesses are closed and schools are closed. Therefore, two of my sisters, two nieces, my daughter, and I are cuddled up with blankets, board games, hot chocolate, and laughter. I enjoy these days although when I have to step outside I often miss my days in Singapore. What a beautiful tropical paradise. The temperatures stay in the mid-eighties although it can rain at any given time. I love the warm rain. My family had wonderful moments I will never forget. This was one of them:

Last week Sophia and I decided to take a trip to the Botanical Gardens. Several people told me there was a wonderful exhibit on biodiversity. The day we decided to go was beautiful. The sky was clear and the sun shining brightly. After a healthy breakfast we headed to the bus stop. There are MANY bus stops in Singapore. It is the primary source of transportation. Once we figured out the correct stop we trekked there. It took about 15 minutes. That's not bad. So what we have done now is sweated out our clothes. We knew the bus would be frigid and we'd dry up. We alighted the bus, got comfortable, and noticed a few drops of rain beginning to splatter across the windshield. That's no big deal; it drizzles often.

Midway through the trip the rain was coming down so hard it looked like someone was standing on top of the bus dumping water over its side. Oh boy. "That's okay," I thought, "we've still got time. And I brought an umbrella. What's wrong with a little precipitation? We won't melt!" When we arrived to the Botanical Gardens 45 minutes later, it looked like it must have to Noah. A rushing river had formed in the street we had to cross. We were determined to go. We had come too far to quit and surely this deluge would end soon. Short bouts of a downpour come and go. We sloshed on, feet soaked through, bent under our teeny tiny umbrella. Inside the gates of the Botanical Gardens we saw a group of elderly people crowding under the one and only covered area available. The path to the food court and exhibit buildings were blocked by police tape. What the heck is going on?! We planned to sit out the storm under cover. There IS no cover! So we cowered under our umbrella on the path hoping for a reprieve. We waited for a half hour. It NEVER let up. We were drenched through from the waist down and starting to shiver. It started thundering and lightning.

We saw a bolt shoot down about a quarter of a mile away. TOO CLOSE! That was it. Time to rush back to the bus, run home and try to savor the silliness of it all. Remember I mentioned the bus being frigid? We FROZE for the entire trip. When we reached our stop and began our mushy walk home, guess what? The sun decided to push the clouds aside. The rain was satisfied that it had replenished Singapore for the day. That's a memory we will take with us from this day on.

Sophia and I eventually made it back to the Gardens and enjoyed its beauty. While I sit here thinking about those days I warm up just a little bit more.

PINK PANTIE
CONFESSIONS

Self-esteem

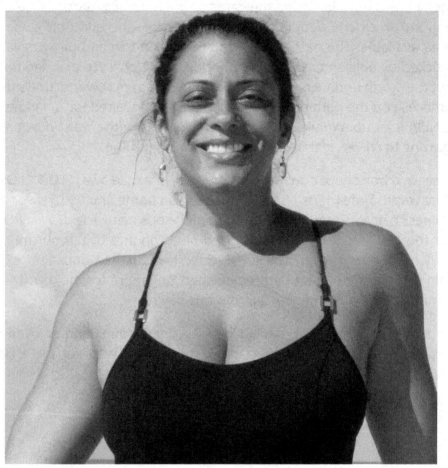

Status:
"I now Choose with Awareness"
April 28, 2014

I love eating at home most of the time. I'm not a bad cook if I put my mind to it, but if I could afford a chef I would have one. My daughter is a picky eater so our meals are pretty simple. Thanks to her dad, she likes food that is good for you. We eat brown rice and beans, salads, greens, steamed veggies, turkey burgers, turkey spaghetti, turkey turkey...Lots of turkey. We also eat some chicken although Sophia can't stand fatty dark meat and refuses anything with bones. She has called herself a "bonetarian" since she could speak. Therefore we tend toward boneless white meat. I have a thing for dark, but why cook it if I'm going to be the only one eating it. We eat fish often (though probably not enough). Sophia's taste runs a little expensive. If she could have shellfish with every meal she would. That ain't happenin'. Not in Chicago. When we lived in Singapore, shrimp, crab, and lobster were inexpensive. Most of the time we would watch as the fisherman would net us out a large crab from the ocean, then cook it right in front of us. I personally can't eat anything that was living seconds before.

I have to admit, I get a little tired of beans, rice, and collards. Every once in a blue moon I don't want to cook! I want to go to a sit-down restaurant. I'm not a foodie, so rarely is the place 5-star. I go to more family-friendly affordable places so we can have our appetizer sampler plate; chicken quesadillas, spinach and artichoke dip with tortilla chips, and hot boneless chicken tenders. Got to have a side salad. Sometimes we'll go for Fajitas... When I'm really being adventurous I'll get a beef cheeseburger. That usually only happens if I need iron. Our favorite place to eat out is Sweet Tomatoes/Soup Plantation. For those of you unlucky enough to not know about this soup and salad buffet, you've got to find one. They are awesome! Going to this smorgasbord has become a family habit. When we get a financial blessing we make our way to Naperville and chow down.

Food used to be my vice. Not good food; no. Nutrition-free food like greasy Chinese and pizza, I used to love it. But my favorite was McDonald's. Yep, I know it's hard to believe. McDonald's. I'd chow down on a double cheeseburger meal with fries and a diet coke. Makes no sense does it? Oh yes it does. When I was a child, McDonald's was our celebratory food. Every two weeks when Mommy got paid we went to Dominic's to grocery shop then McDonald's.

That was the only "restaurant" we EVER went to. It was so much fun. It also gave us a reprieve from my mother's cooking.

I remember when:

We're getting Mickie-Dee's tonight. Cool beans. Haasan's trying to be different, though. He's asking for a icky Big Mac. He never got that before. We always get cheeseburgers and fries -- that's it. That Big Mac is too big! He saw a commercial on TV and said it looks good. I don't think so. Mommy said okay though. Yuck!

I guess it's better than burned chicken wings and string beans or hard pork chops and corn. She tried to make me eat that nasty okra last week. I almost puked. I can't stand anything that feels like snot in your mouth. Daddy wanted chitlins; again. They stink like poop. Eugenia told me that's where they come from – pig intestines. Poop is in intestines. I'm grossing out!! And I'm so sick of kool-aid. We can't ever get pop like everybody else unless we come here to McDonald's. I just love it at this place. It's cool. All my friends eat here whenever they want. They're some lucky ducks.

Haasan starts eating the Big Mac right away cause he's hungry. The special sauce gets all over his face and he is grinning. He says, "I'm a man, now. I'm eating a man-sized burger. Daddy eats these too." He's so funny. Fred, Mommy and I stick with our regular meal. I will never get sick of it. Every two weeks on payday. I love it!

It took me a long time to make the correlation between happy times and McDonald's. Every memorable event in my life was celebrated at McDonald's. Whenever I would get a big job, I'd eat McDonald's. When I found out I was pregnant, McDonald's. Special occasions, McDonald's.

It's funny how our habits are formed in childhood and we don't realize it. I know smokers that can't give it up because their loving Grandma smoked. Some people overeat desserts because their mother made pies, cakes, and cookies on Sundays. Folks don't work out because - "Poppa didn't work out and he lived till 90." People live with depression because - "I can't help it. It runs in my family." Others drink buckets full of alcohol because - "Daddy did it."

Once I recognized my McDonald's pattern for what it was, I began paying attention to all my "bad" habits. I was able to change my life for the better.

For all those who say, this bad habit is 'who I am' I say: You are who you choose to be, from this day forward. You can change your mind about who you are at any given time. Changing our routines start there: Changing our minds. Make a decision then stick to it; then on to the next habit. It is an ongoing challenge. But isn't growth what life is about?

I still take an excursion to McDonald's once in a while. I'll get me a "premium chicken wrap," no sauce, and a small fries. I will also grab a breakfast wrap, orange juice, and coffee in the morning when taking a road trip. I miss my cheeseburgers sometimes. I'm not into denial so if I want one I'll get it. But it won't be because of an internal subconscious urging. I now choose with awareness.

Status:
"I know you love me, as I AM, Baby"
March 3, 2014

Sometimes it seems like the nicest people often end up with not so nice mates. I have had acquaintances and sometimes friends that seem to thrive on the drama of perceived mistreatment. It has driven me crazy over the years when these people I love come to me and complain about how horrible their partner is. I always ask the same question, "Are you sure they're the problem? If so, what are you getting out of it? If you don't like their behavior, why stay?" Really. People invariably do what they want to do. They stay in negative relationships because something within is being fed from the circumstances without. I had a situation once where a friend of mine got in a relationship with someone very close to me. I didn't want to be involved because I saw the potential for disaster. It didn't work. There was pain inflicted. Bitterness bloomed. The sickness of co-dependency sustained until they finally re-alized they were better apart. It wasn't that he was cruel. He just needed more than she would give. He went and got what he needed from someone else, someone that didn't bore him to death. She finally found a man who was happy at home, puttering around the house.

I understand how opposites attract. When two people meet that are worlds apart, everything can seem exciting and fresh. That person will do what you never would. They are loud, you are quiet, they are out-going, you are an introvert, they like to party, you like simple nights with popcorn and TV. You get each other out of your comfort zones. Until you get together long term and those differences start to blow your world apart. Somebody seems like the "bad guy/girl" and the other is the victim. "Why must you drink every day? Why don't you ever want to go out with me? Whose phone number is this? Are you seeing someone else? Do you just want me for my money? You talk too much! You never say anything! You're so dull. You drive me crazy. Stop hitting me. You drove me to it. You are so cold. You are so hotheaded. You'll never change. You'll never change." But they stay even though they're miser-able. That's because they are getting SOMETHING out of it. The problem is, people rarely change.

They are who they are when you meet them. You can't tie yourself to someone for the excitement/peace they bring to your life and then de-cide to change them into your clone when you sign the lease or finalize the marriage license. Either stick with them and love them for who they are, make it work, or get out.

I know You Love Me, as I am, Baby

She laughs in his face
As she sees the look in his eyes
Then walks out the door
"See ya later, lover, I'm going to the store."
But you know she won't be back until about 4... a.m.,
Violet cheeks
Glowing red

As she whispers, "I know you love me as I am, baby. I know you love me as I am."
She falls into a deep sleep
Oh so satisfied
Why are you still there my brother?
Laying by her side?
Does she love you
If she don't treat you like a man?
Like a man
Don't make love no more
Like she used to
Longing, feeling, showing, sharing
Now she just stares at you
Smiling that frozen smile
Going through the motions
Cause you pay the bills
Spending every single solitary dime
She squeezes, and squeezes
Until you cry, my love
You don't know why, my love
You hurt inside, my love
Until you roll up in a ball and die, my love
And Die
She don't love you
If she don't treat you like a man
Like a man
You know she don't
And never will
So get on up
And get on out
Before it's too late
I say, "Man up!"
Get out that deathbed
Jump in that Mercedes car
And dump that witch...
Or stay right there

And love that cheating bitch...

Spoken Word – Cynda Williams; Music – Phil Gardenhire

Status:
Happy 4 the joyous day, Thankful 4 the moment. Grateful 4 abundance.
Now. Today.
March 16, 2014

I had a shock the other day that threw me for a loop. The actual act against me was not important. How I chose to handle the issue was.

So often we are thrown curve balls. Sometimes it's circumstances. Other times it is the people.

I was visiting with a friendly acquaintance of mine about mutual business. While we finished our dealings, he shared with me a recent traumatic experience. Long story short, he had almost lost his life in an accident. He was suffering from post-traumatic stress syndrome. He was having nightmares and anxiety attacks. As he revealed his narrative to me, I noticed that as he told the story, he was reliving the frightening past. He visibly shook and his eyes held terror. I suggested to him that instead of focusing on his near miss, he should instead concentrate on the miracle of his survival. He wasn't ready to receive my proposal. For some reason, he had chosen, for the moment, to be afraid.

As I was caught up in this realization he told me something that blew my mind. Another person had been manipulating my life behind my back. My friend had no idea that what he was telling me was unknown to me. I had an instance where worry and rage threatened to devastate me... Then, I remembered the advice I'd only moments before given him. I understood that I could not focus on the vicious act perpetrated against me. Yes, this supposed friend was trying to throw me into a tizzy. He knew that this acquaintance would share the information. Even with this knowledge, I needed to focus on the now. I was sitting with a kind man, having coffee, and enjoying the beautiful day. The sun was shining and the temperature had finally risen to the 50s. The fear subsided and the anger dissipated. I would have to deal with the new information and the person who had tried to hurt me. I could not be in denial about the need to act, but I could decide right then and there that this untoward behavior against me would not throw me off my cheerful path. In other words, when I finally confronted the jerk I'd be ready. I would not meet him with irate emotional powerlessness; I would stand up to him with an unruffled, sensible demeanor. I would use his strike against him. Not with force but with momentum I created.

We have the power to choose how we view every situation. That is a lesson I have to remind myself of everyday.

OTHER
SHARED CONFESSIONS

JAMES PATTERSON:

First let me say Cynda is a kind, compassionate human being with a great heart. All the things God wants us to be toward one another. Eve-

rything she does in life is done with dignity, class, and courage.

"Your talent, and friendship are extraordinary gifts. And I Thank You for both.

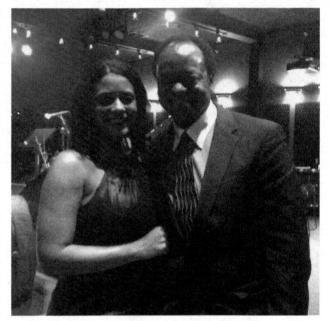

Cynda and James

There isn't a day that goes by that I don't stop and say a prayer for you. I know this book project is a new chapter in your life, and an amazing journey you are embarking on. Thank you for letting me be a part of it. Shine on, my friend..."

-James Patterson

She Will Always Be My Baby

Beverly Williams:

Hello. My name is Beverly Williams. I have so many memories. I don't always know what I learned except that all of it made me stronger.

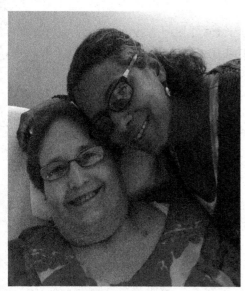

Cynda and her mother Beverly

My father, Albert Leroy Conner, was a beautiful roller skater and diver. That's what attracted my mom, Eula Mae Dennie, to him. He could also ice skate. That's how my parents met; at a skating rink in Selma, IN. They had a sweet romance. My mother was 16 and my father was 18. They courted for two years then got married. I was born two years later. He was drafted into the Army before I was born. My mom was a war bride. Before my father was sent overseas we lived in Tyler, Texas which is not too far from Dallas. He was stationed there. I remember riding the train from Indiana to Texas. My mother got a job as a waitress in a restaurant. It wasn't a good experience. Our home was infested with bed bugs and cockroaches like you'd never believe.

Daddy was ultimately shipped over to Germany. This was World War II. It was bad. He was eventually honorably discharged after he was injured. He had shrapnel in his body, so he was in a hospital for some time. He got a Purple Heart but he killed a lot of people. He brought home stuff, watches (trophies) from those he killed. It affected him. He wasn't the same man. Unfortunately, my father didn't know me. He was close to my younger sister, Kathy. But he was not close to me.

153

Then I got polio at four years old. I remember the night I got it. I don't know what the incubation period was. I remember getting up to go to the bathroom and fell. I couldn't walk. I screamed for my parents. They were asleep. Daddy came and picked me up. I couldn't stand up so they called the doctor in the morning in our town and he came and examined me. He immediately sent me to Riley Hospital in Indianapolis, Indiana. I was there for three months.

That's where I saw my first black person. I had never seen one before and I freaked when the black lady put me in a cart where they take you to a ward. I screamed! I thought later how I must have hurt her feelings. She ended up being the closest friend I had when I was there. When I was four, there was a lot of wrapping legs, warm wraps; that was one of the treatments. They kept these rags in hot water then they would wrap your legs. It was supposed to help. I remember the smell of the rags.

I had several surgeries done there for correction to try to help me to walk for several years. They taught me how to walk with crutches first. I never had full braces because my left leg was always stronger. I had half braces just on my right leg. Later when I got heavier and had children, I had to have full braces.

It was a lot of stress on my parents. I don't know if my father was jealous or what. My mother had to take care of me. My Aunt Margie helped a lot too, but my father didn't seem to like me. He was cold toward me. My parents even thought about going through a divorce but they went to a counselor and decided not to.

It was a very insecure time for me and Kathy. I was six and Kathy was three. I remember Daddy would come and get us when they were separated. It got bad. I had frequent doctor's appointments in Indianapolis. One day my father was angry that my mother was taking me to the doctor. I don't know why he was upset about that, but he was. He had a gun. He fired at us as we were leaving. My mom had to go to one of his brothers-in-law to get some of the tires fixed so we could continue.

I didn't understand because he had taken me to doctor's appointments a lot of times; but he drank. Nobody knows what happens to a man when he goes through a war and has to kill people.

My father did do a lot of great things for me. He taught me to ride a bicycle; he taught me to swim. He let me swim even when I had casts on my legs He'd put me in a big inner tube so I could float around in that. He'd push me. When I had the mumps and couldn't swim, he blew smoke through my ears which would soothe them. He was good in a lot of ways but bad in others.

I understand that he tried the best he could, just like I did. I made mistakes. We all do. I have tried to be the best mother I can. Every birth of all my children (there are five of them) has been different.

It was kind of scary because I didn't really know what to expect. You hear tales, but you never know how hard it can be. My first child's birth is what I want to talk about.

When I was getting near term, I had my sister-in-law, Anna Lee Williams, with me helping take care of me when I moved to Chicago to work. I was in Chicago because the boss I had worked for in college, Dr. Reynolds, called me to work for her in Illinois; the University of Illinois Med Center. Anna came with me to help me during my final bit of pregnancy. She took very

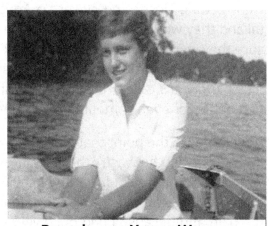

Beverly as a Young Woman

good care of me although we didn't always get along. I'm sure I was testy (I was a frightened pregnant woman) and she always spoke her mind no matter that she might hurt my feelings. I knew she loved me though.

(Cynda's note): What Beverly doesn't say is, she HAD to move to Chicago to work. She was in her senior year of college at Ball State University. She went to work in Anderson at St. John's Hospital doing her work as a medical technologist because they paid a stipend which she needed in order to survive financially. She found out she was pregnant and happily shared the news. Unfortunately, it was against the rules for a pregnant woman to be seen in the hospital working. She thinks the fact that she was married to a black man didn't help her. She couldn't find a job in Muncie.

(Beverly) Dr. Reynolds got me an apartment. The hospital had a residential section. I had no furniture. My mother and father-in-law went out to find me some cheap furniture. We got two couches for sleeping or sitting. We got a couple of nice lamps. I was proud to be able to order an inexpensive beautiful bedroom set and a baby crib.

It wasn't long before I thought that I was having contractions. Anna and I together were timing them. I was setting a time clock. The contractions were getting closer and closer so Anna would take me to the hospital and they would say that I was not in labor. They said I had to make sure they were stronger and to go back home. Anna still tells the story about how we sat and timed the contractions and laughs at me... But I didn't know. It's called "false labor" that many women have with their first babies or even sometimes their other babies.

Finally I got to the point that I KNEW it was real labor. My husband was in the Army (so he wasn't there for me). I started having strong labor. They actually had to induce me once I was in some kind of labor. They made the mistake of giving me a spinal tap or a "spinal" which blocks the pain and because I had polio very young, when I was a child, they could have paralyzed me from the waist down, but God was protecting me and I was young. Cindy Ann Williams was born, although I had named her Rebecca. In my husband's family I had no choices. They named the babies or my husband named the babies. His mother said, "You're not naming that baby after a child in our church!" I thought the child was beautiful and I loved her, but my child became Cindy. (At least) I put my middle name in there – Ann - so she had some part of me.

I was huge as a house. I had put on so much weight. When my husband finally came to see me he was shocked and amazed and told me to "get back in bed."

I couldn't pee and I spiked a fever; a very high fever. They (the medical team) had me sitting in Sitz baths and used all the remedies they had to help you. Of course I had a UTI (urinary tract infection) which is common to me most of my life. Since I had been handicapped for so long I was afraid that something would be wrong with all my babies. We were both anemic but she and I both were fine. I'm just glad she (Cindy) got out safely. She was beautiful. She didn't have a lot of hair so they taped

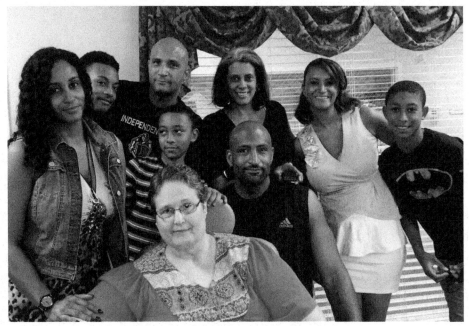

Beverly and her Children

little bows on her head. I was so happy to have her, even though I was sick for some time.

I had a lot of help when I finally did get home. Of course the Williams Family all came. They were so happy to have their second grandchild and that the baby was a girl. They were always a supportive family. My best helper was my brother-in-law James. He took care of me. He would go get baby supplies because at that time, in the 60's, it was taboo to breast feed babies. (We know now) it's the best thing to do.

When I started trying to walk (before my husband went back to duty) he said, "Get back in bed..." He is something else. I loved Cindy and all my babies just like my dad loved me. I think about my mistakes but I try to focus on the good times we had. I am very proud of ALL of them. It upsets me when people spend so much time asking me about my STAR child. They are ALL stars as far as I'm concerned. Cindy was that little pink, bald, bundle before she was on any movie screen. She will always be my baby. I don't care about the rest.

STARTING OVER

ANGIE FORD

I grew up in a Black middle-class residential community in a nice-sized house. As a third generation college graduate, I had most of the things I wanted. I married my college sweetheart. I had a huge wedding with a 28 person bridal party. Over 1,000 people were there! I gave birth to my son nine months after getting married. As a liberal person, I donated to charities and give small change to the needy when I am walking down the street. Three years later, I was a 27-year-old single mother and homeless.

What... the... f*ck?!

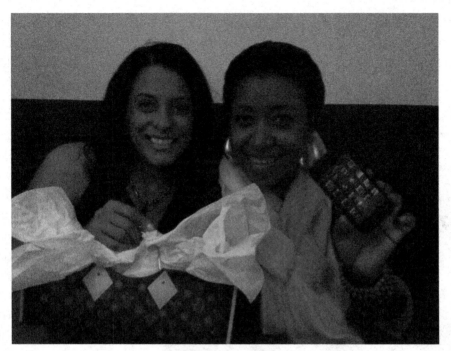

Cynda and Angie

The marriage wasn't working from day one. In college we were two of the most popular people on campus. We enjoyed the notoriety of being a couple and didn't even really consider the fact that we didn't have much in common besides arrogance. Even in the wedding planning, we didn't view money the same. If I hadn't been so caught up in the fact that I was the first of my sorority sisters to get married, I might have noticed this fact. By the fifth month of marriage and the fourth month of my pregnancy, I realized there was no way the marriage would work. Before my son was two, I was so depressed that I was comfortable calling quits on the marriage. We separated and I got my own apartment.

Since I was a freelance artist, I needed to move back home for a few months. Just getting my finances together and finding my own apartment would take a second. I told my Mom and sister that I would be moving back home to the big house (remember?). Well, they told me it would be "embarrassing" to them with the neighbors if I moved back home. After that huge wedding, I would bring them shame by returning home so fast. They told me this in a joint phone call. They were on the landline in the house and I was about to face eviction on the other side of town.

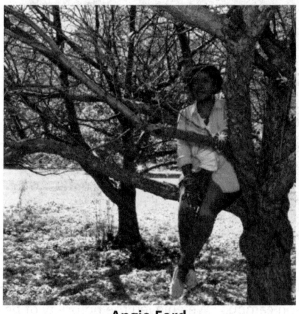

Angie Ford

My son was under three. My grandmother said I could move into her home while she was in Michigan. This gave me a few months; but she was a hoarder, even though no one knew the word back then. Staying in her home was dreadful. She let me move my furniture into her garage that she used for storage. The raccoons and opossums loved it! With no money, I would sleep in a big chair with my feet off of the floor and one eye open while watching over my son laying on the couch. As soon as there was sunlight, I grabbed the stroller and we hit the streets. After 30 days of that, I moved in with my aunt, uncle and cousins. They took me in, as my aunt could not believe her own sister had behaved so awful. My uncle vocally expressed his frustration with having a toddler with poop and diapers in his house. I decided this was absolute bottom.

I decided to be grateful for this moment. I concluded that my son was young, and as long as I presented this as an awesome adventure, he would see it that way. We had our own *"Pursuit of Happiness"* like the movie. It was essential to turning the situation around, mentally heading in another direction. I decided that this mess was the mess that made me more interesting. This story will play out well when I tell my story. Life had been pretty textbook until now and I had not had the opportunity to demonstrate how strong I really was!

When alone in my aunt's basement, I would sit as if in a mock interview with Oprah, as if I were famous and I would describe these dark days. Only then, when I described the termite tunnels boring through the ceiling for the Talk Shows, was it not positively dreadful. The key to the turnaround was when I would describe how this ended in the imaginary interview. I would describe moving out of their basement into this AMAZING apartment with hardwood floors, big windows, where my son had his own room with tons of books and lots of toys. I dared to look for that apartment with the few dollars and awful credit that I had. The story had been told, so that is how it was going to be, right?! I looked at a wonderful apartment. I decided to look fabulous when I toured the place. I was young and well-stacked! I'm not the sum total of my circumstances! When not crying profusely over my situation, I looked GOOD! For this visit, I had on a clingy sweater, a black mini-skirt with opaque black tights and black suede shoes. It was the 90s. "I am an amazing tenant," I told this Brotha, my soon-to-be-landlord. I said, "My credit's crap, but my son is brilliant and he will be starting school right around the block so I will pay my rent!" I made sure I was light-hearted. I locked eyes with him to show confidence, never mind the bead of sweat forming under my bangs. I presented myself as the problem he would NOT have. When I came back to view the place with a security deposit, I bip-bopped around that apartment like a potential prize! I brought my male friend, Bob with me who knew I was trying to close the deal. Bob laughingly asked, "Have you tried sex yet, Angie?!" I laughed and said, "Not yet!" All three of us laughed. But hey, the land-lord let me sign the lease!

I didn't have any furniture. Remember, I gave it to nature's Wild King-dom in my grandmother's garage. My Aunt let me have two old ice cream wire chairs, which I spray-painted. I bought a full-sized mattress and box spring from a local store. My son and I slept together on that mattress the first night. It was one of the best sleeps I ever had. From there, life got really AMAZING! So the story goes...

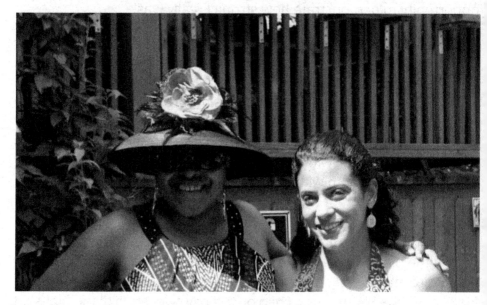

Angie and Cynda

WHEN YOU'RE IN OVER YOUR HEAD

LORRISA JULIANUS:

The toughest chunk of life thus far began when I became the 21-year-old stepmom to a troubled, abused, self-mutilating teen who's own mother had kicked her out just as we got married.

She moved in with us the day we got home from our honeymoon. I had been an over-achieving "perfect child" without teenage friends and could in no way relate to the drama of high school and large-scale rebellion. But I loved my husband for striving to be the best parent he could be, and I couldn't fault him for doing everything to give her the best chance at making it to adulthood in one piece.

Just before then, I'd had a devastating falling out with my greatest emotional support and only immediate family member, my Mom, and I was desperately struggling for work. I learned the hard way that being a published playwright and graduating with a B.A. at the age of seventeen didn't translate into success in the professional world. The expensive court battle with my husband's ex that followed our wedding further added to our stress, followed by a recession and the suicide of my self-employed husband's biggest client. The firm went bankrupt, owing us $25,000. We couldn't refinance our 15-year-loan, couldn't collect unemployment, were forced to work jobs we'd never considered before, depleted our savings, ran up our credit card debt, and had to seriously consider if we should let the house go into foreclosure. All this while having to place locks on our interior doors as we feared for our personal safety.

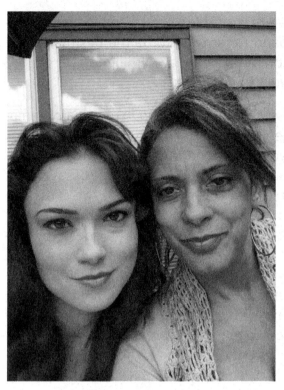

Lorrisa and Cynda

For years we scraped to pay the high bills on the house we bought to shelter ourselves, with an angry, abusive teenager only six years younger than me who had been estranged from us prior to moving in. It sent me back to a time in my isolated, only-childhood when I controlled nothing and lived in constant fear of an angry, alcoholic stepfather. Oh yeah, and the only man I ever called father was found dead about that time. A drunk driver totaled our old car and I ended up with a car payment for the first time in my life.

I had to put down my childhood cat, the only companion I'd had growing up besides my Mom. I adopted another and had to put her down six months later because she had liver failure. I adopted another and had to put him to sleep two months later because he'd gotten feline leukemia from the shelter he was at. My best girlfriend, who had been like a surrogate Mom, died within a day of her cancer surgery. She called me just before she went in, and my last words to Mardee were, "I'm so sorry. I'm starting a gig and can't talk right now. We'll chat after your surgery."

A freak accident left me with a permanent facial scars and a pile of ER and plastic surgery bills. The tenant in our upside-down rental property stopped paying and then started writing bad checks, leaving us on the hook for two mortgages. My husband, my rock through the hard times, was caught between trying to be a firm, loving dad to someone who hated us and saw us as jailers, and doing his best to be an attentive husband who shielded me from her chaos. I wanted nothing to do with the emotionally violent situation and could not face the incredible stress of confronting my stepdaughter on her behavior. He had to do it for me and constantly faced anger on both sides. Meanwhile, this Navy

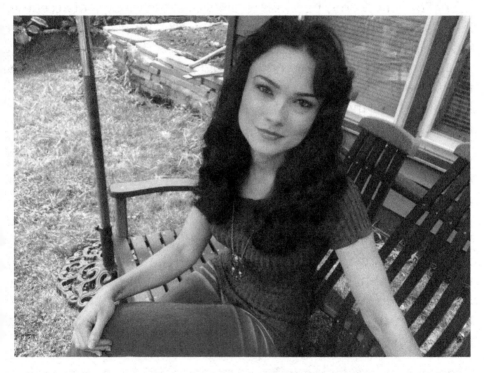

veteran and former SEAL team member who'd ran a successful advertising business for fifteen years couldn't even get a response, much less an interview, to the dozens of positions he applied to online. He was forced to accept work from a questionable former client, which included taking on the man's not-insignificant advertising costs. The client soon stopped paying and had to be taken to court so my husband could collect even part of what he was owed.

Because of the physical toll my anxiety took, including a rare and expensive health condition that caused great pain as well as financial hardship, I went to therapy for the first time in my life, and learned what "boundaries" were. I learned that I didn't have to be a people pleaser, and my needs didn't automatically have to take last place, as I'd always unconsciously believed. Thanks to that therapist, at age 22 I had the strength to turn down a contract for America's Next Top Model when every fiber of my body became literally sick at the thought of accepting it. It was one of the first times I felt empowered for giving a "no" when everything and everyone around me pressured for a "yes." I learned what mindfulness was, and how it could calm my overactive, anxious mind. I learned that taking care of myself and being the best me I could be, before I was the best stepmother or wife I could be, would spill over in positive ways to the rest of my life.

My performing work had dried up to nothing with the recession, and I decided on a whim to begin painting just because I wanted to. Without a day of art lessons, I was displayed in my first gallery within two months and today I pay my bills comfortably as a sought-after artist. Through an extremely odd modeling gig I acquired and managed to get my husband hired on as well. He met the person who, two years later, recommended him for his current position, which has changed our lives and given us an even better life than we had before the recession. Our savings have been restored, and I'm in better shape and health than I was a decade ago.

I continue my exploration of meditation, mindfulness, and modern spirituality, and have channeled my discoveries and journey into writing that has changed the lives of people suffering with the same anxieties I faced. My stepdaughter is a beautiful, successful, happy young woman today, and we are closer than I even dreamed possible. I learned a Buddhist teaching and experienced its truth – nothing lasts forever, neither good nor bad.

As each year stretched on, it seemed that our debt and stress and horrible jobs would never end, but they did. Not only did that give me perspective and appreciation for my blessings today, but every skill I learned and honed in that time created the reality I'm living today - personally, professionally, and spiritually. Without the loss of his biggest client, a difficult firm that did its best to bully and low-ball him, my husband would have never found his dream job.

I cultivated lifelong friendships that I never would have known without those game nights at home because we were too broke to go anywhere. I'm still less than thrilled at the prospect of confrontation, but I no longer accept abusive behavior just to avoid having to say to someone's face, "What you are doing is not respectful or acceptable and I need you to stop." I have learned to speak my mind clearly and calmly in such situations, and I no longer feel the rush of adrenaline with trembling hands, pounding heart, and a fight-or-flight response. It's a skill that came later than others and with many bumps, as tolerating everything in silence was the only acceptable response during my childhood. I am less concerned with winning approval from people I can't even respect, and I more easily recognize the best way to handle a negative situation. Now I can say to myself, "Hell, I've been through a lot worse. This is a piece of cake." And surprise, surprise - taking the risk pays off and the person in question doesn't key my car, egg my house, get me blackballed, or throw a screaming tantrum after all. I learned sympathy and solidarity with those who suffer with financial hardship, physical trial, grief, or family abuse and rifts. Those tough years taught me that money isn't everything.

Outside adversity forged my marriage like steel that had been through the fire and came out stronger. We recognized that every trial we faced wasn't between us; it was from the world around us, and that drew us closer as we depended even more on each other. And I learned that I was more powerful than I thought I was. I also recognized that my struggles, such as they were, were nothing compared to the physical, mental, and emotional suffering endured by millions of women worldwide or down the street. I always enjoyed a loving, supportive marriage to my best friend, clothes on my back, food on the table, and never feared death by illness or at the hands of another person. So many of my friends survived sexual and physical assault, multiple cancer diagnoses, devastating divorce, and still kept their smiles, their attitude of gratitude, and refused to see themselves as victims. Those women are my heroes.

Mine is not a fairy tale ending – my life is just getting started and isn't perfect – and the changes for the better didn't happen overnight. But when I think back on those years, the biggest stressors of today grow a little lighter. I'm more grateful for those things I took for granted before – my physical health, living pain free, my mental health, my restored relationship with my Mom, my husband's happiness in his job, my cats' health, a roof over my head that we can pay for without worry. I'm more grateful for the little luxuries we couldn't dream of then – organic produce, a dinner out, a new article of clothing, a vacation, being able to afford petunias for the flower beds, not having to panic at an unexpected maintenance bill. I'm grateful for the many, many friends I have now that I didn't have when I got married. Back then I could have counted my real friends on one hand with fingers to spare. And in the darkest moments, at my wit's end, trying to please my industry's professionals who didn't care about me, when I was fighting for every role and opportunity that then fell through, I was so tired of being a pawn with no say over my life or career. I had to find a personal dream to cling to again.

I hadn't written in years. The only dream I could find that stuck was from childhood and was the most improbable of all. I dreamed of writing the book and lyrics to an epic musical about Zenobia, the ancient warrior queen of Syria. I dreamed of becoming the strong, unstoppable Zenobia, on a grand, romantic scale that would blow away everything I'd ever seen onstage. I didn't know how it could possibly happen but I decided to write it anyway, holding that dream close to my heart and nurturing it day after day, month after month.

With seventy friends at my side, that show premiered four years later. The newest of those friends was a woman named Cynda Williams. I knew nothing about her other than that she was a talented performer, volunteered to work backstage, and was a warm, dependable person I wanted to learn more about. Because of Zenobia, I've continued writing and sharing stories of suffering and joy, of inner strength and the power of love. The more time that passes, the further those hard, un-ending times recede into memory. And they will for you too. You may feel like a bloodied warrior fighting hand to hand in a battle that never ends. But it will end. Everything does. You may not get to decide if you walk away with a handsome scar or have to be carried off the field with a leg missing, but you get to decide the person you'll be because of it. Will you be a victim of war or a triumphant hero? Breathe. Smile. This is just the beginning.

Lorrisa is a published playwright and SAG-AFTRA actor with credits that include WB's DC Comics videogame, Injustice: Gods Among Us, the Mortal Kombat franchise, The Lord of the Rings Online, and guest appearances on The Bold & the Beautiful for CBS and Chicago PD for NBC. Her second language is Middle Egyptian, and her dream is to host and write a historical travelogue series. She and her husband Craig have been together since 2005, and are certified crazy cat people. Lorrisa graduated with a Screenwriting B.A. from Columbia College Chicago as their youngest graduate at age 17, and had her first full-length script published by an imprint of Samuel French when she was 16. Her historical plays have been produced as far away as Moscow, and her internationally exhibited fine art can be viewed at the Facebook page "The Art of Lorrisa Julianus, 'Embrace the Night.'" Clips from her musical, Zenobia, can be viewed at youtube.com/zenobiathemusical, and performance rights are available. Her latest play, Made of Stars, premiered in spring 2015 and is a journey through the three incarnations of seven souls across two millennia. Six-time Emmy winning writer Kay Alden called it "A sweeping saga through time and cultures, raising issues of spirituality, mortality, and the power of love. A charming, entertaining, yet deeply thought-provoking drama."

A GIRL SOLDIER'S STORY

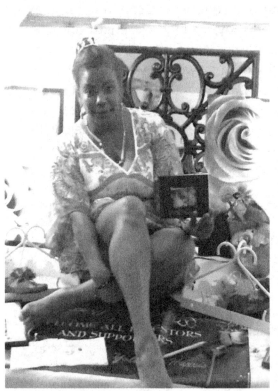

Yolanda Harris

YOLANDA HARRIS:

I knew you as Cindy Williams. To say Cynda sometimes, I trip over and go, "Hmmmm, Cynda." That's what everybody else knows her as. I know Cindy. I know her so closely that at school one day I accidently gave her some medication that made her sick, so her acting career began with me acting like I was sick (and her going along with it) so we could both go home together cause I thought I killed my best friend.

We went through Bennet all the way through eighth grade. We had a lot of fun at Bennett. I mean we would have this game we played called, "Johnny Run Across." (*Laughing*) The boys would be on one side - and the girls - they would try to catch us. Then we had this game called, 'Catch a Girl, Kiss a Girl.' Nobody wanted to play that game. You know, there was a guy named Grady; I ended up kicking him and the next day he transferred out of the school. Cynda had her love affair with a big red-haired boy that just was her 'daallll" baby.

We used to sit there in her room painting fingernails and would sit on her porch on 104th and King Drive and eat and talk. There was a lot of bonding with each other. The summer after (our) graduation my dear friend left me and moved to Muncie, IN. That was a pinnacle moment in my life: to lose a best friend... I didn't see her in high school and then she went off to college.

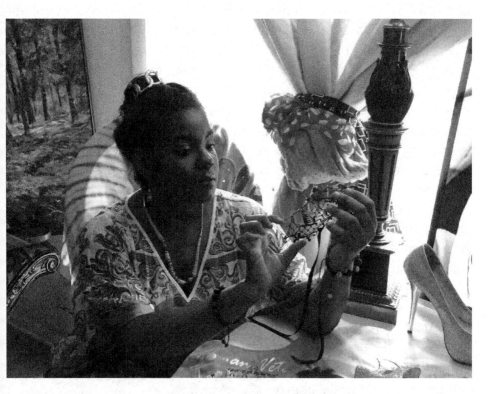

After I went to Tuskegee Institute, I immediately joined the military. When you remove yourself from who you're really close and connected with, you try to search for that connection again. When I went to the military I tried to form some friendships, some strong bonds because in the military you have this bond that you have to go through in boot camp. Our boot camp company was very integrated. They purposely made it integrated. We had 11 white Caucasian females and 10 Black females. They gave us a flag that was supposed to be called "K111."

When we looked at it, it was the 'Kill' company. We figured out that it was an experimental company; they were experimenting by putting half black and half white in this company.

I ended up getting into a fight while in boot camp and I've never fought in my life. Back in Bennett, a girl chased me across ice and snow and chipped my tooth because I would run away from fights. But I had never been called a racial epithet at home in Chicago before. To be in the military and to be called a racial epithet was just really strange. Everybody said, "Oooo...You're going to let her get away with that..." So I ended up getting into a fight with this lady. She was from Oklahoma so she LARGER than I was; probably four inches taller and about forty pounds heavier. Well we fought. We got sent to something called intensive training. They exercise you till you fall out and faint. Well, while we were exercising I'm steady trying to hold her up so she wouldn't fall and faint and afterwards she asked me, "Why would you do that after I called you a nigger?" I said, "It wasn't about that. It was about me not being alone

having to do all this exercise; so I had to keep you going." And she said, "You know, that's what teamwork and a partnership is about." So the rest of boot camp, and the time we were there, we all stuck very close together. We won every award they had. We got the 'Cinderella' liberty which allowed us to stay out an hour more after graduation. Our boot camp made history. They never had another K111 squad again after that.

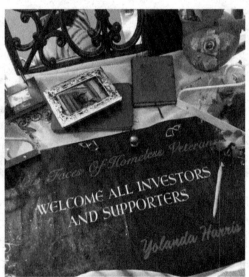

Yolanda's Non-for-Profit

I was an overachiever; I was always trying to do everything to the utmost, so they changed my job from electrician aircraft mechanic to weapons. I didn't know what that meant at the time. I went through all of the self-paced learning; electronics school, weapons school, parachute school, and special marksmanship. They gave me my orders and, me being a city girl, looked at the orders and said, "These orders say, Pascagoula, Mississippi." I didn't think that was possible. Pascagoula, Mississippi? I said, "I'm only eighteen years old and I gotta go to Mississippi? No!"

I get to the ship and this is the first time I had ever had a panic attack. I saw this humongous ship in dry dock on stilts. You could see the ship from the bottom all the way to the top. We had to climb this scaffolding up to the ship. Based on Navy protocol you have to salute the flag before you enter the ship. I was so nervous, I felt like I was about to pee on myself. To put it plainly, I was just scared.

After I got on this ship, they had this Marine come and get me from the ship of interest and take me down to the weapons department. Not only did I have to walk across this humongous ship, I had to walk down into the bowels of the ship. I'm like, big doors clanging, big turns, big handles; it was just something... your eyes are like forty inches big looking at this. You're like a small kid, eighteen years old, never been on a ship and like, "what have I gotten myself into?" I get on the ship. They tell me I'm in the Weapons Six Department.

Weapons Six Department is Special Weapons which means you're security over the entire ship. You're over the MPs. You're the one that is responsible for the nuclear conventional weapons, the hand guns, everything. I wasn't prepared for that. On top of all that, I was the only female...

Yolanda Harris is very active with women veterans. She has helped many find peace after tormenting experiences in the military. She has her own not-for-profit organization named 'Women Veterans Apparel' (WVA). Most veteran apparel is geared toward men, as if the women that serve are insignificant. WVA designs clothing just for female vets. WVA also supports other non-profit organizations focused on assisting female vets.

Yolanda continues telling her intriguing yet horrifying story of survival in "Pink Pantie Confessions – Bringing the Hot Pink Back into the Royal Blue."

***

YOU ALWAYS SEE THEM SMILING

LYNNE HATFIELD:

Hi, my name's Lynne. When I met Cindy it was because I had to do her hair and makeup for a poster. She was advertising Dreamgirls at the Muncie Civic Theater. We had a mutual friend, Todd, who asked me to do it. The only thing was, the night before I had to do her hair and makeup, my husband confessed to me that he was having an affair with his skanky secretary. The next day I was upset and crying... It was horrible but I had to show up and meet Cindy. I believe that God put her in my life at the

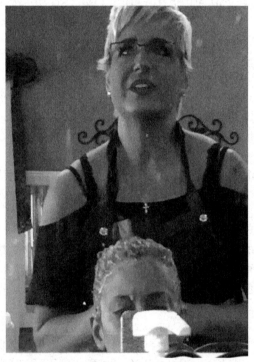

Lynne doing Cynda's Hair

174

worst time in my life. We ended up becoming fast friends. She slept in my guest bedroom while she did the play and helped me through a really horrible time in my life. She had been staying in an apartment at The Civic which was beautiful but fortunately for me she was allergic to mold and was unable to stay.

Cindy staying with me and is probably one of the reasons why I continued to work out my marriage with my husband. She made me see things in him that I didn't see or even want to see...so...I'm still married. That was two years ago.

My confession has nothing to do with my husband (who I love very much in spite of the troubles we had) and our problems and survival. He is my second husband. My earlier life was very different. My first marriage was terrible. I worked at this big fancy salon; probably the best salon here in Muncie. I got pregnant. I didn't want the baby. When the baby, Hayden, was born and he had something wrong with him, I was absolutely devastated. I felt guilty. He was autistic.

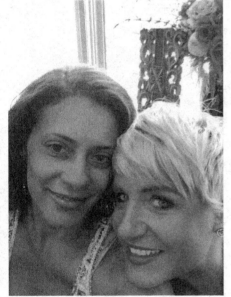

Cynda and Lynne

Raising a child with special needs, I never realized... I mean you don't plan on having a child with special needs. You never think about that when you're growing up or plan on that. You never realize the difficulty parents with special needs have from the outside looking in. I mean, when Hayden needed to get his hair cut he'd throw fits. Children with autism don't like being touched. They have sensory issues. I had to go into the salon after it was closed because he'd throw such a fit it would take three of us to hold him down.

175

People stare. When we go out in public we always had to apologize to people. They judged us and still do. You're always making excuses...you feel bad...It's just so...so sad. I hated always saying, "I'm so sorry, my son's autistic." I hated making excuses for him when around people...I don't comprehend why they can't be understanding about it. The older Hayden got, the worse it got.

One experience really opened my eyes. One Christmas when Hayden was older, he wanted to go see Santa Claus. Most of the people in line were little kids. Hayden was probably a sophomore at Southside. I don't know...but he was obviously the oldest kid in the line. He was so nervous about seeing Santa. He kept saying, "Mommy, Mommy, I don't know what I'm gonna say. Mommy I don't know what I'm gonna ask for!" I was like, "I don't know. You just need to tell him." We got to see Santa and he was so excited about that.

We started walking around the mall for a little bit. I stopped by a place that sells jewelry and boots. I was bedazzling boots that year so I walked in. The rest of the family stood outside the store waiting for me. There

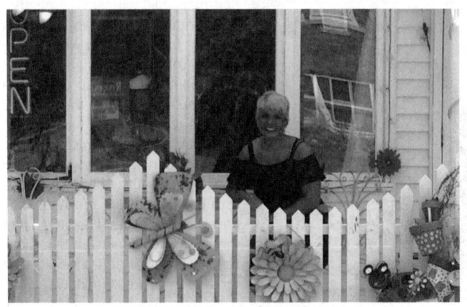

Lynne in Front of Her Shop

were these high school girls standing there. I leaned across them to see what the price was on these boots and this high school girl goes, "Oh my God, there's that retard. He's following us!" She was just saying all this stuff about Hayden and I just froze. I was like, deep inhale... I can't believe they're talking about my kid! I was just like... I couldn't believe it! I just didn't know what to do. I was... that Mamma Bear came out of me. The girl was talking on her phone and said, "We were there watching the little kids talk to Santa and this retard, ugh!" She was saying all this stuff! I was just fuming! I looked to see and make sure she was talking about Hayden. She was talking about Hayden! She dropped her phone and I picked it up and I said to the girl on the line, "You really need to question who your friends are. You really do." I handed the phone back to the girl. I said, "You're talking about my son. He's not following you, he's with me." She said, "I'm not talking about your son!" I pointed at Hayden and said, "You're talking about MY son." They may have been middle schoolers. I said, "The fact is that he's smart enough not to be a horrible person. Retard is a horrible word. He was excited to see Santa Claus. You just took a wonderful night and ruined it by being a little bitch." I don't know what else I said. I just saw red and my mouth took over. The lady with the store came up asking if there was a problem. I said, "Yes...This girl is horrible." My husband Bobby (current husband) came in to get me and dragged me out. Hayden said, "It was me Mommy wasn't it? She was mad at me. She was mad at me." I said, "No. She was just a stupid little girl. It's totally fine." But I really was shaking and mad and crying. I was like, "Why can't there be a place where these kids are accepted and wanted and don't have to explain themselves? Why are people so stupid?" I was so mad. People are like this.

Eventually Bobby took me to a book store where they have coffee. He sat me down and said, "We're going to have to get you a catch phrase or something." By then I had gone off on people before. He said, "Things happen and you have to have something to say to them." So he got me these cards that explained how my son was autistic and what that meant. That was supposed to help me not go off on people. That was fine; but you know on the back I had printed, "and piss off." I think it's

177

terrible we have to give cards to people to explain why our special needs kids are the way they are. The rest of us should understand.

I wanted a place that parents could come and bring their kids to cut their hair. We (here at Simply Beautiful) as hair stylists know what to do to make it easier for them. They don't have to say, "I'm so sorry. My son is autistic or has Downs." Or whatever... They don't have to feel ashamed. They don't have to feel anything. If we have to get down on the floor and roll around with them to cut their hair, we do; anything. They can cry and

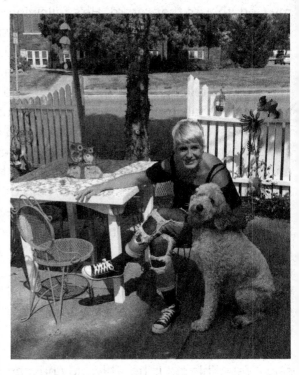

they can scream and they can wipe snot on us, whatever... It's okay. None of us here care. They are accepted. They are wanted. They are loved. I can't tell you how many parents have sat here and cried because they love it. We've gotten so many letters. I understand how that feeling is because I've been there. I've been where they are.

It's not special needs people that need to change; it's us that needs to change. We need to learn to be accepting. They are angels here on Earth. Their skies are always blue. It's us that have the issues. I would love to live in their world. You always see them smiling.

CPSIA information can be obtained
at www.ICGtesting.com
Printed in the USA
FSOW03n2310300516
20978FS